ADVANCES IN PHYSIOLOGICAL SCIENCES

*Proceedings of the 28th International Congress of Physiological Sciences
Budapest 1980*

Volumes

1 – Regulatory Functions of the CNS. Principles of Motion and Organization
2 – Regulatory Functions of the CNS. Subsystems
3 – Physiology of Non-excitable Cells
4 – Physiology of Excitable Membranes
5 – Molecular and Cellular Aspects of Muscle Function
6 – Genetics, Structure and Function of Blood Cells
7 – Cardiovascular Physiology. Microcirculation and Capillary Exchange
8 – Cardiovascular Physiology. Heart, Peripheral Circulation and Methodology
9 – Cardiovascular Physiology. Neural Control Mechanisms
10 – Respiration
11 – Kidney and Body Fluids
12 – Nutrition, Digestion, Metabolism
13 – Endocrinology, Neuroendocrinology, Neuropeptides – I
14 – Endocrinology, Neuroendocrinology, Neuropeptides – II
15 – Reproduction and Development
16 – Sensory Functions
17 – Brain and Behaviour
18 – Environmental Physiology
19 – Gravitational Physiology
20 – Advances in Animal and Comparative Physiology
21 – History of Physiology

Satellite symposia of the 28th International Congress of Physiological Sciences

22 – Neurotransmitters in Invertebrates
23 – Neurobiology of Invertebrates
24 – Mechanism of Muscle Adaptation to Functional Requirements
25 – Oxygen Transport to Tissue
26 – Homeostasis in Injury and Shock
27 – Factors Influencing Adrenergic Mechanisms in the Heart
28 – Saliva and Salivation
29 – Gastrointestinal Defence Mechanisms
30 – Neural Communications and Control
31 – Sensory Physiology of Aquatic Lower Vertebrates
32 – Contributions to Thermal Physiology
33 – Recent Advances of Avian Endocrinology
34 – Mathematical and Computational Methods in Physiology
35 – Hormones, Lipoproteins and Atherosclerosis
36 – Cellular Analogues of Conditioning and Neural Plasticity

(Each volume is available separately.)

ADVANCES IN
PHYSIOLOGICAL SCIENCES

Satellite Symposium of the 28th International Congress of Physiological Scienc
Visegrád, Hungary 1980

Volume 27

Factors Influencing Adrenergic Mechanisms in the Heart

Editors

M. Szentiványi
A. Juhász-Nagy
Budapest, Hungary

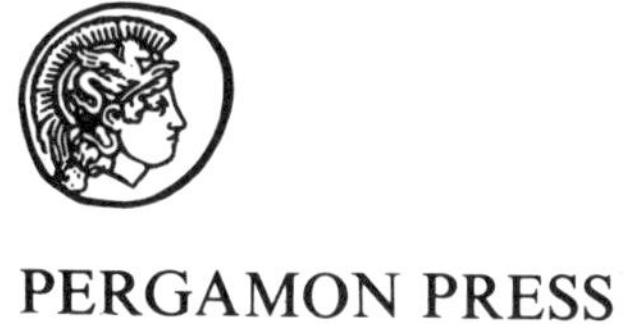

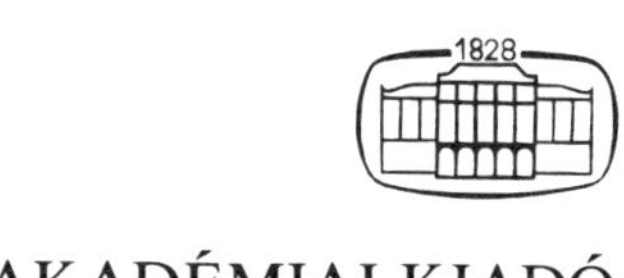

PERGAMON PRESS   AKADÉMIAI KIADÓ

Pergamon Press is the sole distributor for all countries, with the exception of the socialist countries.

HUNGARY	Akadémiai Kiadó, Budapest, Alkotmány u. 21. 1054 Hungary
U.K.	Pergamon Press Ltd., Headington Hill Hall, Oxford OX3 0BW, England
U.S.A.	Pergamon Press Inc., Maxwell House, Fairview Park, Elmsford, New York 10523, U.S.A.
CANADA	Pergamon of Canada, Suite 104, 150 Consumers Road, Willowdale, Ontario M2J 1P9, Canada
AUSTRALIA	Pergamon Press (Aust.) Pty. Ltd., P.O. Box 544, Potts Point, N.S.W. 2011, Australia
FRANCE	Pergamon Press SARL, 24 rue des Ecoles, 75240 Paris, Cedex 05, France
FEDERAL REPUBLIC OF GERMANY	Pergamon Press GmbH, 6242 Kronberg-Taunus, Hammerweg 6, Federal Republic of Germany

British Library Cataloguing in Publication Data

International Congress of Physiological Sciences
   Satellite Symposium (28th : 1980 : Visegrád)
   Advances in physiological sciences
   Vol. 27: Factors influencing adrenergic mechanisms
   in the heart
   1. Physiology - Congresses
   I. Title   II. Szentiványi, M
   III. Juhász-Nagy, A.
   591.1   QP1   80-42203

Pergamon Press	ISBN 0 08 026407 7 (Series)
	ISBN 0 08 027348 3 (Volume)
Akadémiai Kiadó	ISBN 963 05 2691 3 (Series)
	ISBN 963 05 2753 7 (Volume)

In order to make this volume available as economically and as rapidly as possible the authors' typescripts have been reproduced in their original forms. This method unfortunately has its typographical limitations but it is hoped that they in no way distract the reader.

Printed in Hungary

CONTENTS

PREFACE

This volume contains the papers presented at one of the satellite symposia of the 28th International Congress of Physiology.

The past few years have witnessed numerous new achievements that modify the traditional views of adrenergic regulation of cardiac muscle and coronary blood vessels. These achievements tended to diversify immensely the technical detail of our knowledge about the intricate mechanisms involved in heart activity. At the same time, despite their ramifications, these results can be classified into two main groups characterized by different intellectual climates: one which stems from Langley's concept of cellular "receptive substances" and finds its fullest expression in dogmatic forms of receptor theory; the other which stresses the chemical environment rather than the structural characteristics of the regulated myocardial elements and stems, essentially, from the Bernardian concept of "milieu interieur". The organizers of this symposium think that an unnatural conceptual separation of the two great fields of inquiry took place: the study of receptors and that of the modulating humoral agents; and although in the present state of research, there are unmistakable trends of a desire to break down the articifial barrier between them, still one must admit that as yet too little has been accomplished towards effecting this end.

Such reflections have led us to organize the symposium. It would have been a mistake, on the other hand, to make its goal too encyclopedic or pedantic. Instead, the authors were encouraged to present their own opinion and speculations, and — in general — to give their work a more "personal flavor" than it is usually customary in scientific articles.

We do hope that the symposium will generate as much new research as it attempted to cover.

Finally, we should like to express our gratitude to our colleagues and co-workers, Miss Viola Kékesi and Mrs Vera Németh (National Institute of Vascular Surgery, Budapest) as well as to Mrs Csilla Kiss, Miss Mária Pénzes and Miss Ágnes Paál (Chemical and Pharmaceutical Works, CHINOIN) for their invaluable help with organizing the meeting, proof-reading, checking of problems and index.

M. Szentiványi
A. Juhász-Nagy

WELCOMING ADDRESS

> "Research is to see that everybody has seen
> but to think that nobody has thought"
>
> (Verulam Bacon)

Ladies and Gentlemen,

You certainly know the famous maximum of Verulam Bacon "Research is to see that everybody has seen but to think that nobody has thought". Let me start with the analysis of this motto.

The first part of the statement "Research is to see — something that everybody has seen" means that everybody may see what he wants, nobody can be deterred from seeing truth. However, the second part ". . . but to think that nobody has thought" is more important because seeing leads to thinking, and thoughts cannot be hindered by the outside world we are living in.

Only if the thoughts of scientists are free can bring seeing (that everybody has seen) to the action of mind; to think that nobody has thought.

Thus our motto leads us to the freedom of sciences. Everybody has to fight in his own environment for this freedom. You have to fight for peace because "Inter arms silent Musae", also the muse of science.

If somebody from the side of power says: "Be on our side", you should stop seeing. However, scientists accustomed to use their brains fro seeking truth. No matter what kind of power wants them to be blind, they cannot be cheated. Anything false, aggressive or oppresive must be fought by men of science who know that seeing is not enough, thinking is also needed.

If we now scrutinize the realm of adrenergic reception, two major areas will be taken into consideration: two ways of truth. One was found by Cannon and Rosenblueth. They approached the path from the side of transmitters. The question to be answered was why the adrenergic response is different in various areas. For this reason they stimulated the nerves of different organs and recorded the effects on other remote fields, in so-called test organs. Since the same vegetative organs were influenced differently when the sympathetic nerves of various remote organs were stimulated they concluded in the difference of mediator substances released. A release of mediator + an inhibitory substance (Sympathin I) or an excitatory substance (Sympathin E) was postulated to explain adrenergic inhibitory and excitatory effects.

Another explanation was based on the existance of different kind of receptive substance. These different adrenergic receptors should be responsible for the ambivalent effects of catecholamines (Ahlquist).

In the first case the response of a substance would have been demonstrated at the transmitter level. Although the humoral effects could not be denied, the theory of Cannon and Rosenblueth was rejected simply because they were unable to demonstrate the existance of I and E Sympathins.

Ahlquist's theory, on the other hand, could not reply the questions and explain the facts of the humoral hypothesis: Why and how different reactions will be elicited on the same test organs by stimulating different sympathetic nerves? Finally, how can different humoral pathways make rendered possible different effects?

It seems to be two sides of one truth. Our motto should be altered accordingly: Truth is not what we see but that we can think of. Neither the humoral nor the receptor theory is valid or both are. In the latter case, a third theory or new facts must be added.

I hope that at this symposium at least some new facts will emerge even if no comprehensive theory can develop. Looking forward to reaching this goal, have all the participants my best whishes.

M. Szentiványi

EFFECTS OF ADRENALINE ON SOME ASPECTS OF ELECTRICAL AND MECHANICAL ACTIVITY IN THE FROG HEART

G. Vassort and R. Ventura-Clapier

*Laboratoire de Physiologie Cellulaire Cardiaque, FRA 51 INSERM, Bât 443, Université Paris-Sud,
F-91405-Orsay, France*

Myocardial behaviour is known to be altered by catecholamines. In the following the effects of adrenaline were investigated on three aspects of frog heart mechanical activity : increase in the slow current and related mechanical strength 1) in normal medium or 2) in metabolic-deficient solution and 3) increase in the rate of relaxation of tension. These aspects are considered significant examples of three major topics in the excitation-contraction coupling of the heart muscle cells : the amplitude of tension is controlled by the free intracellular Ca concentration but also by the energy-rich phosphates available at the myofilament sites ; besides, the relaxation is dependent upon the rate of decrease in intracellular Ca following its uptake by the internal sites or extrusion through the cellular membrane.

The experiments were performed under voltage clamp conditions on frog (Rana esculenta) atrial trabeculae, 70-150 μm in diameter, by means of a double sucrose gap method with simultaneous recording of mechanical activity (Vassort and Rougier, 1972). Tension was measured in the test compartment with a transducer element (serie AE 800 from AME) lengthened by a thin lever (4 cm long ; 50 mg weight).

Effect of adrenaline in normal medium

Two different inward currents are responsible for the development of the cardiac action potential. The Ca current may be distinguished from the initial Na current in several ways since the conductance mechanisms involved respond differently to drugs and since they have different dependences on potential and time. The initial current is completly inactivated by holding the membrane at -40 mV and is inhibited by tetrodotoxin (TTX) ; in both conditions a Ca current may be elicited by applied depolarizations.This latter current is inhibited by Mn or La ions and by verapamil or D 600. The rather slow inactivation time course suggests that the Ca conductance contributes to determine the duration of the action potential. The correlation between Ca current and tension is striking in the frog heart (Fig. 1). Tension increases rapidly when the Ca current first become appreciable. The peak tension

1

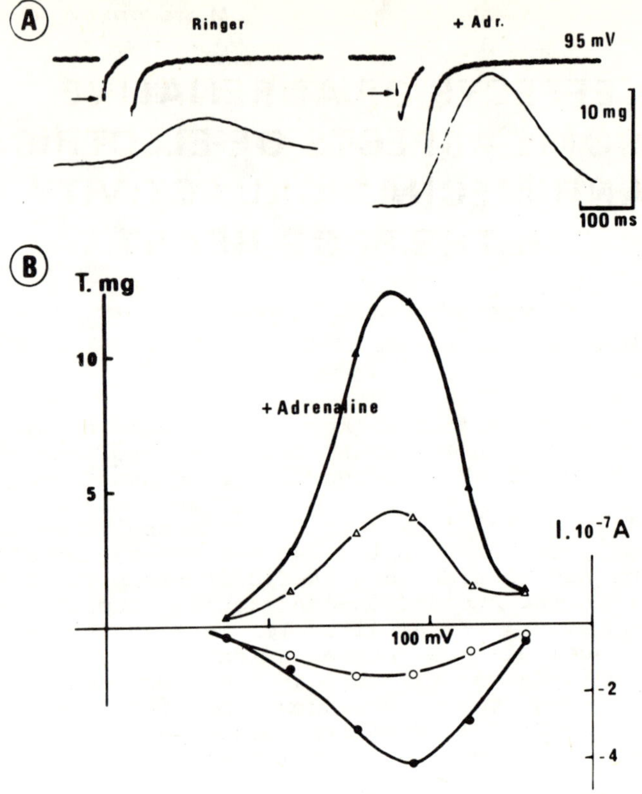

Fig. 1 : Effects of adrenaline (5×10^{-6}M) on the slow Ca
inward current and the phasic tension. A : for a given
depolarizing step (95 mV-60 msec), adrenaline increases both
the slow inward current (upper traces) and the mechanical
activity (lower traces). The fast Na inward current is
unchanged (arrows). B : peak tension and maximal inward
current plotted against the depolarization applied to the
membrane from its resting potential (E_r) in Ringer solution
(open symbols) and after the addition of adrenaline (closed
symbols) (Vassort, 1973).

occurs at the same potential as for peak Ca current and, when
the membrane is further depolarized towards the Ca equilibrium
potential both Ca current and tension decline. However when
pulses longer than the 50 msec used here are applied, a
second component of tension is elicited that is independent
of Ca current. It increases with the amplitude of the depolarization and with the duration of the pulse up to about
1 second. This component of tension accounts for the fact that
tension is maintained as long as depolarization is. This latter
component was named "tonic tension". The first one, dependent
on the Ca current, is refered to as "phasic tension"

(Vassort and Rougier, 1972). These two components of tension
are also evidenced in mammalian heart (Coraboeuf, 1974). Tonic
tension was recently shown to depend on the Na-Ca exchange
mechanism located at the cellular membrane (Horackova &
Vassort, 1979).

A further correlation between Ca current and phasic
tension was provided by the effects of adrenaline. In addition
to its chronotropic action in heart, adrenaline increased the
force of contraction. Adrenaline has been found to increase
the Ca current inflow (Vassort et al., 1969, Reuter, 1974).
It also increased markedly the peak tension elicited by short
depolarizations (Fig. 1). Both increase in current and tension
occurred simultaneously with a half-time about 1 min. On
the other hand, tonic tension did not seem significantly
altered by adrenaline.

<u>Effects of adrenaline during CN-poisoning</u>

During CN poisoning, oxidative metabolism is impaired.
This leads to a decrease in mechanical and electrical
activities on which the ability of adrenaline to counteract
the inhibition was tested.

On frog heart, cyanide produces an initial rapid decrease
in peak tension followed by a decrease in action potential
duration and amplitude (Fig. 2). Once tension was reduced to
20 % of its initial value, adrenaline (10^{-6}M) allowed only
incomplete recovery of maximal tension whereas action potential
amplitude was enhanced. Such weak effects of adrenaline has
been also described for mammalian heart under hypoxia
(Davidson et al., 1974).

The same events were analysed in voltage clamp experiments.
In cyanide, the two components of tension, phasic and tonic
were decreased within 5 min prior to alteration in the Ca
current. After 15 min both Ca current and tension were
diminished to a steady value. When adrenaline (10^{-6}M) was
added, it produced a large and rapid increase in Ca current
to about four times the peak current in Ringer solution while
tension recovered nearly its initial value (Fig. 3B). The
graph in Fig. 3A gives both the peak tension and peak current
elicited by 60 mV-160 ms pulses (holding potential -40 mV)
in order to differentiate the time courses of the rises in the
slow inward current and tension induced by adrenaline
(5×10^{-7}M) in the presence of cyanide. It is noticeable that
the time courses of both increases are very different. Peak
inward current increased very rapidly with a half time of
about 20 sec while the increase in tension appeared to be
delayed and slow (half time : 90 sec). Such different time
courses between electrical and mechanical activity following
the addition of adrenaline has been shown in the hypodynamic
frog heart (Niedergerke and Page, 1977).

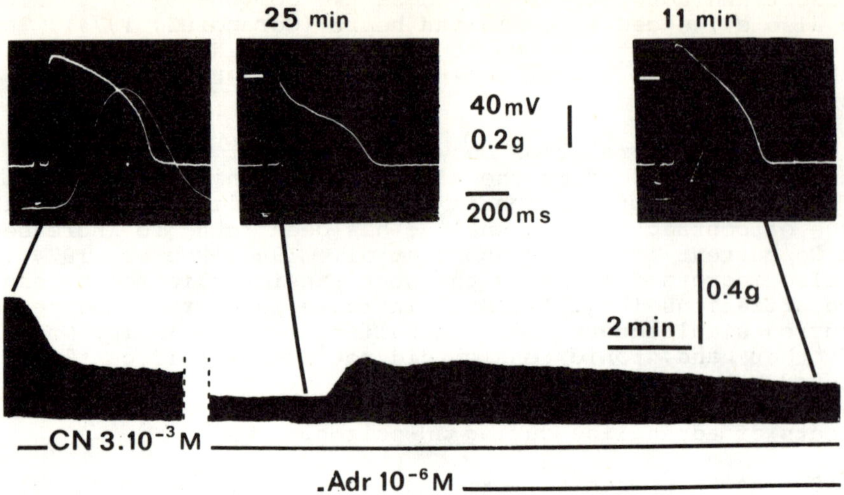

Fig. 2 : Effects of adrenaline (10^{-6}M) in the presence of cyanide (3×10^{-3}M) on the electrical and mechanical activities of frog heart. Upper traces : action potentials and tension recordings before and after 25 min in cyanide and a further 11 min in cyanide plus adrenaline taken from a representative experiment. Notice the recording was stopped for 14 min during cyanide application.

These results suggest that the effects of adrenaline on tension depend on the metabolic state of the heart. Although Ca current was largely increased in the presence of both cyanide and adrenaline the increase in tension was delayed and not in proportion with the increase in Ca current. A dissociation appears between the two events and must be accounted for by an other mechanism regulating the amplitude of tension. Cyanide poisoning induces a large decrease in creatine phosphate whereas ATP concentration is not signi-ficantly altered (Ventura-Clapier and Vassort, 1980), suggesting a regulatory role of creatine phosphate for tension development, creatine phosphate being the metabolite shuttling between the energy synthesis sites and the energy utilization sites. Such a primary role of creatine-creatine phosphate has been recently reviewed (Saks et al., 1978). The dissociation between electrical and mechanical events following adrenaline suggests that adrenaline was not able to counterbalance mito-chondrial poisoning induced by cyanide and to restore the initial CP level. The results reinforce the existence of a dual control of mechanical activity by Ca and energy-rich phosphates located at the myofilaments sites.

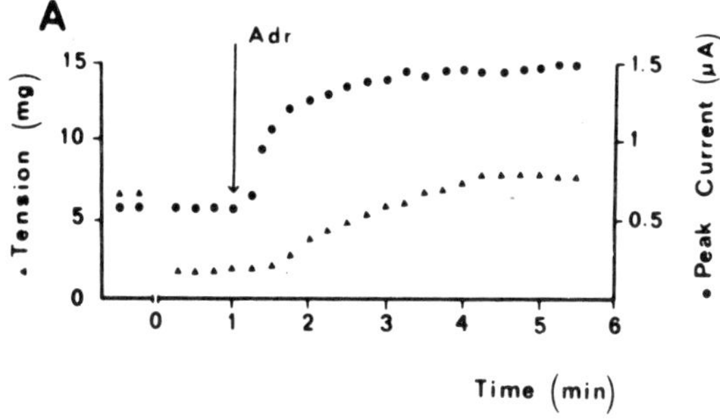

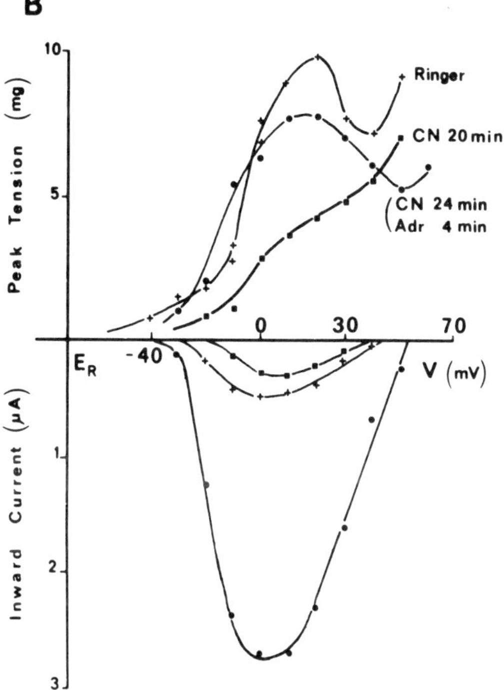

Fig. 3 : Analyses of current and tension under voltage clamp conditions. A The peak slow inward current (filled circles) and peak tension (filled triangles) elicited by 160 ms - 60 mV pulses (with a holding potential : E_r + 30 mV) are plotted versus time to differenciate the time course of rises in current and tension after application of adrenaline (5 x 10^{-7}M). The first two points show the amplitudes in normal Ringer. Zero time is taken as 7 min after the addition of cyanide. B Slow inward current and peak tension-voltage relationships illustrating the effects of adrenaline (5 x 10^{-7}M) in the presence of cyanide (3 x 10^{-3}M)(filled circles). Curves for normal Ringer (crosses) and after 20 min cyanide (filled squares) are reported.

5

LA RAIA, P.J. & MORKIN, E. 1974. Adenosine 3', 5'-monophos-phate-dependent membrane phosphorylation. A possible mechanism for the control of microsomal calcium transport heart muscle. Circ. Research, _35_, 298-306.

MEINERTZ, T, NAWRATH, H. & SCHOLZ, H. 1975. Relaxant effects of dibutyryl cyclic AMP on mammalian cardiac muscle. J. Cyclic Nucleotide Res., _1_, 31-36.

MORAD, M. & ROLETT, E.L. 1972. Relaxing effects of catecho-lamines on mammalian heart. J. Physiol., _224_, 537-558.

NIEDERGERKE, R. & PAGE, S. 1977. Analysis of catecholamine effects in single atrial trabeculae of the frog heart. Proc. R. Soc. Lond. B., _197_, 333-362.

REITER, M. 1972. Differences in the inotropic cardiac effects of noradrenaline and dihydroouabain. Naunyn-Schmied. Arch. Pharmac., _275_, 243-250.

REUTER, H. 1974. Localization of beta adrenergic receptors, and effects of noradrenaline and cyclic nucleotides on action potentials, ionic currents and tension in mammalian cardiac muscle. J. Physiol., _242_, 429-451.

ROULET, M.J., MONGO, K.G., VASSORT, G & VENTURA-CLAPIER, R. 1979. The dependence of twitch relaxation on sodium ions and on internal Ca^{2+} stores in voltage clamped frog atrial fibres. Pflügers Archiv., _379_, 259-268.

SAKS, V.A., ROSENSHTRAUKH, L.V., SMIRNOV, V.N. & CHAZOV, E.I. 1978.Role of creatine phosphokinase in cellular function and metabolism. Can. J. Physiol. & Pharmacol., _56_, 691-706.

TSIEN, R.W. 1977. Cyclic AMP and contractile activity in heart. Adv. Cyclic Nucleotide Res., _8_, 363-420.

VASSORT, G. 1973. Existence of two components in frog cardiac mechanical activity. Influence of Na ions. Europ. J. Cardiol. 1/2, 163-168.

VASSORT, G. & ROUGIER, O. 1972. Membrane potential and slow inward current dependence of frog cardiac mechanical activity. Pflügers Archiv., _331_, 191-203.

VASSORT, G., ROUGIER, O., GARNIER, D., SAUVIAT, M.P., CORABOEUF, E. & GARGOUIL, Y.M. 1969. Effects of adrenaline on membrane inward currents during the cardiac action potential. Pflügers Archiv., _309_, 70-81.

VENTURA-CLAPIER, R. & VASSORT, G. 1980. Electrical and mechanical activities of frog heart during energetic deficiency. J. Muscle Research & Cell Motility (in press).

DISCUSSION

<u>Rubányi</u>: Do you think that the transmembrane ion transport is supplied mainly by ATP produced by glycolysis?

<u>Vassort</u>: In fact, it appears so; probably because the energy consumption of membrane ion transport is low, the ATP production by glycolysis is sufficient for it. It is not sufficient, however, for the high energy demand of the myofilaments.

<u>Szentiványi</u>: In our experiments in which we are showing the existence of a new substance that can regulate ATP pathways we have also shown that calcium-deficiency is also influenced these pathways. If, in the frog heart, we poison the ATP generation with dinitrophenol /DNP/, our "regulatory substance" can reestablish the blocked mechanical activity /contractions/. On the other hand, if the frog heart was inhibited by calcium-free Ringes solution, it movements came also back when the heart was treated with this substance. It was followed that Ca receptors and ATP cycle had to be near to each other.

<u>Vassort</u>: Such neighboring points can be imagined.

<u>Juhász-Nagy</u>: I think Dr. Vassort summerized brilliantly the multiple actions of adrenaline on excitation-contraction coupling in the heart. Another question is the <u>modulation</u> of the effects exerted by the catecholamines under different circumstances. Adenosine, e.g., an important modulatory substance has little or no effect on mechanical or electrical activity of the ventricular muscle, although it is very potent in producing other effects such as bradycardia and coronary vasodilation. However, adenosine is not a negative inotropic effect in an ordinary sense of the word: the nucleoside does not even decrease much the augmented ventricular contractility produced by exogenous catecholamines, as Szentmiklósi has conclusively shown it /Szentmiklósi et al., this symposium/. /Acetylcholine which is another "indirect" negative inotropic agent in the <u>mammalian</u> heart was shown to affect primarily the catechol-stimulated ventricular muscle./ The modulatory role of adenosine on ventricular myocardium is necessarily linked to two alternative mechanisms or conditions which are not mutually exclusive. One of them is the presynaptic inhibition of neuro-effector transmission. Dr. Szentmiklósi and I, independent of each other, came to this conclusion, and both of us will speak, later on, about the mechanism of it. The other condition is the quality of action potential in the ventricular muscle. If you inactivate the fast Na^+ conductance by K^+-induced depolarization, the heart stops but could be reactivated by catecholamines. In this case the electrical /and mechanical/ activity becomes dependent upon the secondary inward current carried by Ca^{2+}. The above type of reactivation, at the same time, is paralleled by the appearance of the sensitivity toward adenosine, i.e. the direct modulation of adrenergic effects by adenosine occurs only in the presence of a Ca-dependent action potential.

We suppose that precisely the same thing could happen in the
human heart after an ischemic episode, when the extracellular
K^+ is elevated and the heart is under a strong adrenergic drive.
Adenosine, also released by the hypoxic myocardium, may be a
dominant agent in modulating heart activity. This is, of course,
pure speculation, and whether this really occurs in myocardial
infarction, we don't know. But we know that this mechanism ex-
its in the human heart in the operating theatre. Dr. Valeria
Kecskeméti, while working in our laboratory, has shown that
after a cardiac operation with cardiopulmonary bypass, ventricular trabeculae taken out of patients subjected to temporary
myocardial ischemia and K^+ /the principal ingradient of the so-
-called protective solutions in cardiac surgery/ adenosine de-
presses the contractile force and inhibits the action potential.
In the normal human heart it does not produce such an effect.
Essentially all these are connected to the unusually strong
Ca-dependence of cardiac activity.

Rubányi: In supporting this conclusions I should like to men-
tion that Ca^{2+} current is preferentially inhibited by adenosine
in the isolated coronary artery as shown by Harder and his co-
-workers. /Harder et al.: Circ. Res. 44: 176, 1979/

HEART RATE CHANGES IN NEUROGENIC HYPERTENSION

Eduardo M. Krieger, Elisardo C. Vasquez and Alceu S. Trindade, jr.
*Department of Physiology, Faculty of Medicine of Ribeirão Preto, U. S. P. — 14.100 Ribeirão Preto,
S.P., Brazil*

Neurogenic hypertension has been produced in several mammalian species
by radical denervation of the sino-aortic baroreceptor areas (for references, see McCubbin and Ferrario 1977). More recently, an increase in
sympathetic output was obtained by central deafferentation of the baroreceptors as a consequence of localized brainstem lesions (Nathan and Reis
1977). Baroreceptor-denervated animals show great blood pressure lability
under different behavioral conditions, but the average 24-hour mean
arterial pressure appears to be less altered (Cowley et al. 1973). In the
rat, when the anatomical peculiarities were identified (Fig. 1) and the
sino-aortic afferent fibers were cut, chronic neurogenic hypertension was
also obtained (Krieger 1964).

This procedure to produce sino-aortic denervation in the rat has been
used successfully in several laboratories (Thant et al 1969, Jones and
Hallbäck 1977, Chalmers et al 1979, Alexander et al. 1980). When direct
mean arterial pressure was measured in unrestrained conscious sino-aortic
denervated rats for only a short period of time (15 minutes), hypertension
of more than 150 mm Hg was observed, even after one year of denervation
(Krieger 1964). In a more recent study (Krieger and Trindade 1980), when
arterial pressure was measured continuously during a 16-hour period the
average increase was less than that observed for short period measurements;
the average increases were 37 ± 9, 27 ± 10 and 16 ± 7 mm Hg, respectively,
after 1, 7 and 180 days of denervation.

No marked tachycardia was detected in rats with neurogenic hypertension
in the hemodynamic studies performed on conscious animals immediately
following denervation and 6 months after operation (Krieger et al. 1979).
As seen in Fig. 2, mean arterial pressure rose 30% above control values 1,
5 and 6 hours after denervation. The cardiac output measured in conscious
rats by the thermodilution technique actually decreased, with the rise in
peripheral resistance being the only factor responsible for hypertension.
The drop in cardiac output was caused by reduction in stroke volume
(0.091 ± 0.010 vs. 0.115 ± 0.005 ml/100 g) with no additional increase in
heart rate after denervation, since the control value was already high
(478 ± 9 vs. 455 ± 7 beats/min).

Hemodynamic parameters analyzed 6 months after bilateral sino-aortic
denervation showed that hypertension still persisted and was maintained
exclusively by increased peripheral resistance, with cardiac output
remaining normal. The heart rate of the conscious neurogenic hypertensive
rats during hemodynamic analysis was similar to that of the normotensive

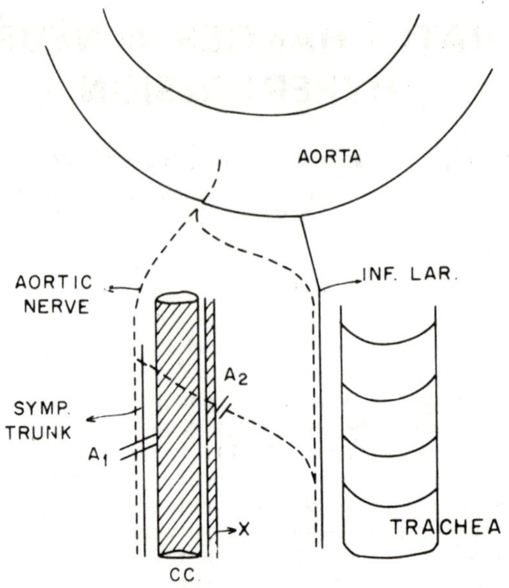

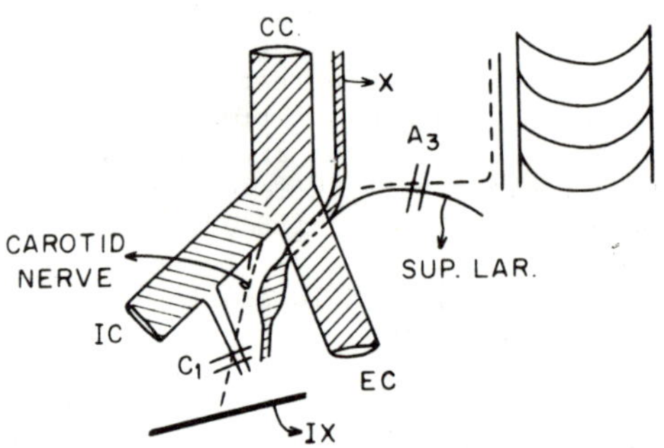

Fig. 1. Schematic presentation of baroreceptor distribution in the rat, with indication of the sites where the aortic (A_1, A_2, A_3) and carotid (C_1) fibers are cut.

rats (435 ± 14 vs. 434 ± 9 beats/min). Therefore, the fact that no tachycardia was previously detected in neurogenic hypertensive rats could be attributed to the control heart rate values that were extremely high (about 400 beats/min). However, as shown previously (Soato and Krieger 1974), when the heartbeats were measured by means of the ECG obtained from chronically implanted electrodes rather than by arterial pressure pulses,

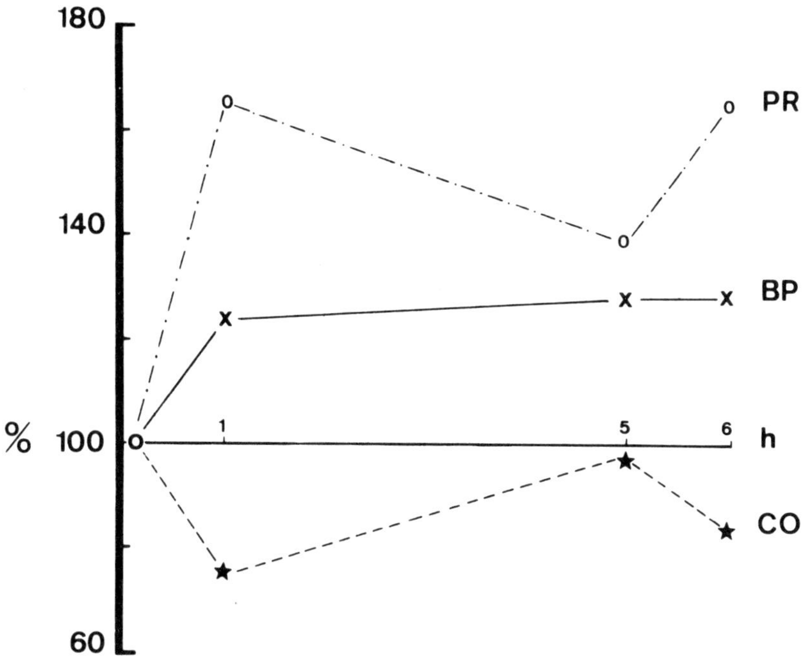

Fig. 2. Changes in blood pressure (BP), cardiac output (CO) and peripheral resistance (PR), expressed in percentage, following sino-aortic denervation in 9 unanesthetized rats. CO was measured by the thermodilution technique.

the heart rate was considerably lower (about 320 beats/min), indicating that the rat also has a predominantly vagal tone under resting conditions. Using this technique, we can see a progressive tachycardia after sino-aortic denervation reaching its maximum after 5 hours of denervation (Fig. 3). In previous studies on rats, maximal elevation in arterial pressure was observed within the first hour after denervation (Krieger 1970, Krieger et al. 1979, Doba and Reis 1973), the same as observed in cats, which showed an increase in pressure occurring more rapidly than tachycardia following lesions of the nucleus tractus solitarii (Nathan and Reis 1977). Isolated denervation of the aortic baroreceptor produced a tachycardia quite similar to that exhibited by the rats subjected to total denervation (Fig. 3), while isolated sinus denervation produced only a mild increase in heart rate. These data indicate that in the rat there is a predominance of the aortic over the carotid depressor fibers in the regulation of the resting heart rate, the same predominance of the aortic baroreceptors described previously for regulation of arterial pressure (Krieger 1964, 1970). This is in contrast to the data usually reported for dogs (see Donald and Edis 1971); however, recently the preferential importance of

the aortic receptors in setting the mean level of arterial pressure has
also been emphasized in dogs (Ito and Scher 1979).

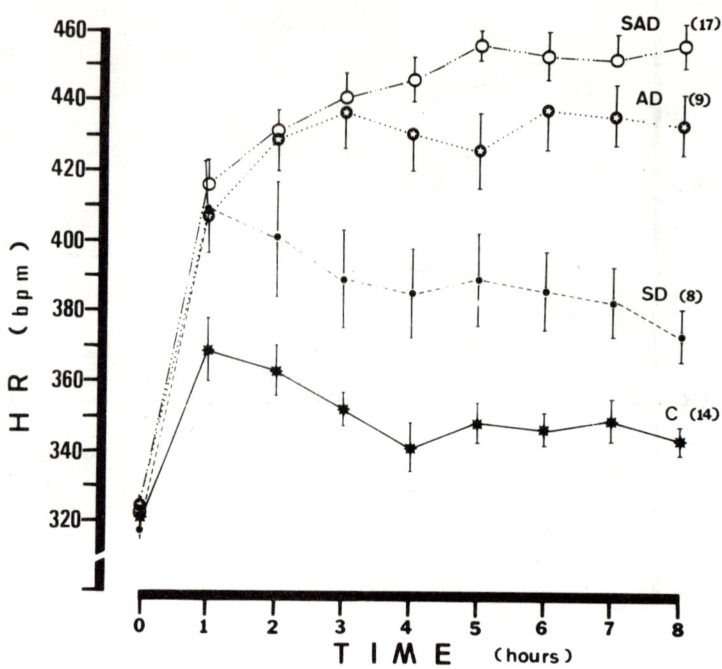

Fig. 3. Evolution of resting heart rate after cessation of ether anes
thesia for baroreceptor denervation: isolated sinus denervation (SD),
isolated aortic denervation (AD), total sino-aortic denervation (SAD)
and sham-operation (C). Mean ± S.E.

The tachycardia seen under resting conditions in the acute phase of
neurogenic hypertension (Fig. 3) was not maintained and progressively
declined. Even in the rats subjected to bilateral sino-aortic denervation
daily measurements showed that heartbeats had returned to normal values
(337 ± 6 beats/min) 10 days after surgery. Following transitory tachycardia and 3 days after normalization of the resting heart rate, a continuous recording of the arterial pressure over a period of 6 hours to minimize excitation showed that the sino-aortic denervated rats were still
hypertensive (141 ± 5 vs. 113 ± 6 mm Hg for the control rats). An indication that the procedure used for pressure measurement did not overesti-
mate the pressure values, due to excitation of the rat, is the fact that
the basal resting heart rate calculated by the pressure pulses was not
different from that obtained by the ECG in the undisturbed animals (347 ±
6 vs. 327 ± 11 beats/min). The data for the first time indicate a complete
resetting of the heart rate after radical denervation of the baroreceptors.
In a study on conscious rabbits subjected to total sino-aortic denervation,
Alexander and De Cuir (1970) reported that 2 to 5 weeks were required for

14

the heart to slow down to about 50% the initial increase, though complete
resetting rarely occurred within this time.

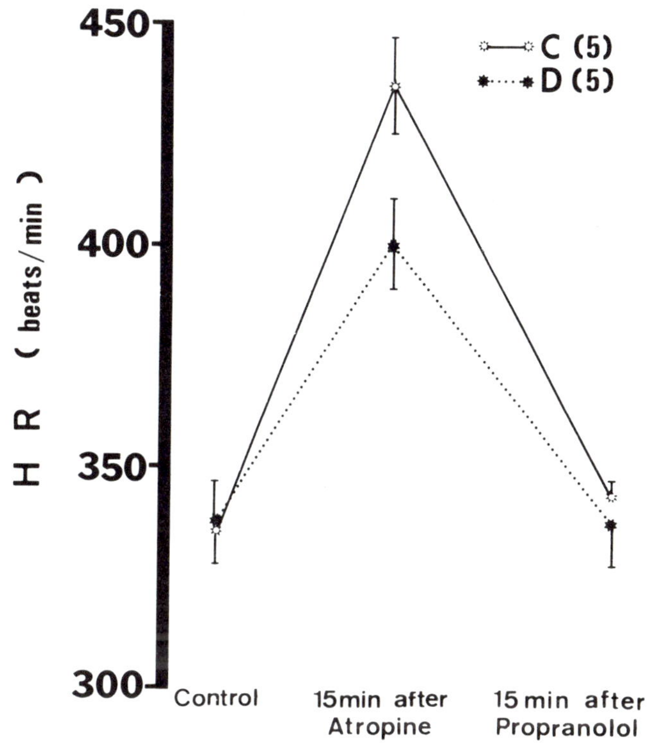

Fig. 4. Heart rate responses to atropine followed by propra
nolol in conscious control (C) and conscious sino-aortic de
nervated rats (D) 3 days after normalization of the heart
rate. Mean ± S.E.

Sympathetic and vagal tones were assessed in conscious rats by autonomic blockade produced by intraperitoneal injection of atropine (4 mg/kg)
and propranolol (6 mg/kg). To avoid excitation during injection the drugs
were administered through a thin silastic tube implanted into the abdo-
minal cavity. Intrinsic heart rate measured after blockade with atropine
plus propranolol was 5% lower in the conscious hypertensive rats 3 days
after recovery from tachycardia than in the control rats (327 ± 7 vs. 350 ±
4). The rats with normalized heart rate had a 40% smaller increase in
heartbeats after atropine than the normotensive controls (Fig. 4). The
decreases in heartbeats produced by propranolol (Fig. 5) were significantly smaller in the denervated rats than in the controls when compared with
the intrinsic heart rate (10 ± 1 vs. 46 ± 5 beats/min) but not when compa

red with the control heart rate (20 $\pm$ 8 vs. 32 $\pm$ 6 beats/min).

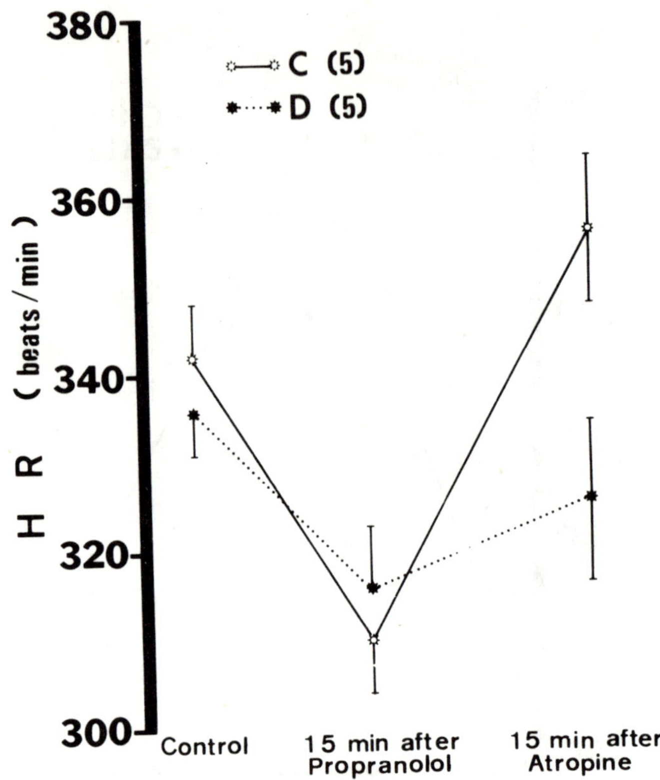

Fig. 5. Heart rate responses to propranolol followed by atropine in conscious control (C) and conscious sino-aortic denervated rats (D) 3 days after normalization of the heart rate. Means $\pm$ S.E.

The decrease in vagal tone after transitory tachycardia in the sino-aortic denervated rats is not surprising since the baroreceptors normally stimulate the vagus. Unexpectedly, these rats exhibited a decreased sympathetic tone, which may be related to the mechanism causing reversal of tachycardia even when hypertension is maintained. There are indications in the literature that increased sympathetic traffic to the heart can induce a decrease in responsiveness to β-adrenoreceptor stimulation (Fujiwara et al. 1972, Lowe 1974, Julius et al. 1975). In another series of experiments, we observed that the neurogenic hypertensive rats with normalized heart rate had hyposensitivity of the heart rate to infusion of progressive doses of isoproterenol and to stress stimuli. The decrease in heart rate sensitivity to sympathetic activity, possibly associated with a central

resetting of the reflex arc that regulates the sympathetic tone for the
heart, could account for the recovery from tachycardia after baroreceptor
denervation even when hypertension persisted.

SUMMARY AND CONCLUSIONS

When the heartbeats of the rat are measured by ECG through chronical
ly implanted electrodes the resting heart rate is quite low (about 320
beats/min) indicating a predominance of the vagal tone. Total denervation
of the sino-aortic areas produced a marked tachycardia reaching its maximum within 5 hours. Isolated denervation of the carotid and of the aortic
fibers indicated that the aortic baroreceptors play a predominant role in
heart rate regulation in the rat, as previously observed in a study on
blood pressure regulation. Tachycardia progressively declined and the
resting heart rate returned to normal in 10 days after total aortic
denervation when the rats were still hypertensive. When the denervated
rats were submitted to autonomic blockade with atropine and propranolol
3 days after recovering from tachycardia, their intrinsic heart rate was
lower and their sympathetic and vagal tones smaller than for the rats with
intact baroreceptors.

(Financial support by FAPESP and FINEP. Technical assistance by E.D.
Moreira and A.A. Maia).

REFERENCES

Alexander, N., Velasquez, M.T. and De Cuir, M. 1980. Indices of sympathe-
    tic activity in the sinoaortic denervated hypertensive rat. Am. J.
    Physiol. 238: H 521 - H 526.
Alexander, N. and De Cuir, M. 1970. Heart rate resetting after partial or
    total sinoaortic denervation in conscious rabbits. Am. J. Physiol. 219:
    107-113.
Chalmers, J.P., Petty, M.A. and Reid, J.L. 1979. Participation of adrener-
    gic and noradrenergic neurons in central connections of arterial barore-
    ceptors. Circ. Res. 45: 516-522.
Cowley, A.W., Liard, J.P. and Guyton, A.C. 1973. Role of the baroreceptor
    reflex in daily control of arterial pressure and other variables in the
    dog. Circ. Res. 32: 564-576.
Doba, N. and Reis, D.J. 1973. Acute fulminating neurogenic hypertension
    produced by brainstem lesions in the rat. Circ. Res. 32: 548-593.
Donald, D.E. and Edis, A.J. 1971. Comparison of aortic and carotid barore-
    flexes in the dog. J. Physiol. 215: 521-538.
Fujiwara, M., Kuchii, M. and Shibata, S. 1972. Differences of cardiac
    activity between spontaneously hypertensive and normotensive rats. Eur.
    J. Pharmacol. 19: 1-11.
Ito, C.S. and Scher, A.M. 1978. Regulation of arterial pressure by aortic
    baroreceptors in unanesthetized dogs. Circ. Res. 42: 230-236.
Jones, J.V. and Hallbäck, M. 1977. Cardiovascular reactivity and design
    in rats with experimental "neurogenic hypertension". Acta Physiol. Scand.
    102: 41-49.
Julius, S., Randall, O.S., Esler, M.D., Kashima, T., Ellis, C. and Bennett,
    J. 1975. Altered cardiac responsiveness and regulation in the normal
    cardiac output type of borderline hypertension. Circ. Res. 36-37, Suppl.
    I: I-199-I-207.
Krieger, E.M. 1964. Neurogenic hypertension in the rat. Circ. Res. 15:
    511-521.

Krieger, E.M. 1970. Acute phase of neurogenic hypertension. Experientia
   26: 628-629.
Krieger, E.M. and Trindade Jr., A.S. 1980. Long-term analysis of neurogenic hypertension in the rat. Proc. Intern. Union Physiol. Sci. XXVIII
   Intern. Congress - Budapest 14: 530.
Krieger, E.M., Moreira, E.D. and Silveira, M.F. 1979. Hemodynamic studies
   in conscious neurogenic hypertensive rats. Jap. Heart J. 20, Suppl. I:
   68-70.
Lowe, R.F. 1974. Sympathetic induced alteration in cardiac function in
   baroreceptor inactivated dogs. Clin. Res. 23: 5A.
McCubbin, J.W. and Ferrario, C.M. 1977. Baroreceptor reflexes and hypertension. In Hypertension (Ed. J. Genest), McGraw-Hill Book Company, New
   York, pp. 128-133.
Nathan, M.A. and Reis, D.J. 1977. Chronic labile hypertension produced by
   lesions of the nucleus tractus solitarii in the cat. Circ. Res. 40: 72-
   81.
Soato, G.G. and Krieger, E.M. 1974. Heart rate after acute hypertension
   in the rat. Am. J. Physiol. 227: 1389-1393.
Thant, M., Yamori, Y. and Okamoto, K. 1969. Baroreceptor function revealed
   by acute sinoaortic denervation in spontaneously hypertensive rats. Jap.
   Circ. J. 33: 501-507.

DISCUSSION

- Dr. Juhász-Nagy: Did the plasma epinephrine level increase? During the
  hypertensive period (denervation) other reflexes originating from the
  heart may take over heart rate regulation?

- Dr. Krieger: Circulating levels of catecholamines were measured by Dr.
  Alexander (Alexander et al. 1980) when studying the sympathetic activity
  indices after sino-aortic denervation in the rat; she found increased
  plasma NE and E within the first 3 weeks after denervation. Regarding
  your second question, in a preliminary study in our laboratory, bilateral vagotomy performed 6 days after sino-aortic denervation produced an
  additional increase in pressure, suggesting that the vagal afferent
  nerves from the cardiopulmonary region may play an important role in
  blood pressure regulation in the absence of the influence of the arterial baroreceptors.

- Dr. Rubányi: Did you measure any parameter of myocardial contractility
  or metabolism? The possibility exists that arterial receptors take over
  the regulatory role of denervated high pressure baroreceptors. What are
  your comments about this possibility?

- Dr. Krieger: No, we did not measure myocardial contractility or metabolism in neurogenic hypertensive rats. Regarding your second question, we
  have already mentioned to Dr. Nagy that in the rat also, as shown for
  cats, rabbits and dogs, the vagal fibers from the cardiopulmonary areas
  could have a moderate inhibitory effect on the sympathetic outflow that
  regulates blood pressure. However, we have not tested the influence of
  these receptors on heart rate regulation.

- Dr. Szentivanyi: In normal animals we see fluctuations of blood pressure
  and heart rate and these fluctuations increase after NE administration.
  So the changes are very complicated.

18

- Dr. Krieger: There is general agreement that after baroreceptor denervation (peripheral or central deafferentation) the animals exhibit a
great arterial pressure and heart rate lability. The major role of the
baroreceptors seems to be counteracting the fluctuations of the circulatory system under the different behavioral conditions. The extent of
mean arterial pressure increase over 24-hour periods of observation is
still being debated. When evaluating the increase in mean blood pressure
level after sino-aortic denervation the following considerations are
relevant: the animal species used, the extent of baroreceptor denervation, the time elapsed after denervation and, especially, the various
behavioral conditions during blood pressure measurement.

- Dr. Kunos: We made a similar observation of β-adrenergic hyposensitivity
in SHR rats (published in Life Sci. 1978).

DEVELOPMENTAL CHANGES OF THE CATECHOLAMINE-INDUCED CHRONOTROPIC RESPONSES OF CHICKS RELATED TO THE BLOOD PRESSURE RESPONSES

G. Rabloczky and M. R.-Mader

Institute for Drug Research, Budapest, Hungary

The aim of this study was to observe the maturation of heart rate responses upon adrenaline administration in chicks of several ages. The earliest age was the 10th–11th day of incubation, the latest one was the "adult hen", i.e. more than three months old after the hatching.

Methods

a/ Chick embryo experiments
After removal of the eggshell on a small field, one branch of the main umbilical artery going to the chorioallantoic membrane was cannulated by a rather thin polyethylene catheter. This canule served for arterial pressure measurement. Concomitant smaller vessel coming from the chorioallantoic membrane's vascular network /umbilical "vein"/ was also cannulated for intra venous drug administration. The position of the inserted canules are schematically demonstrated on Fig. 1.

By means of this method the measurement of the blood pressure and heart rate of chick embryos could be performed without the use of any anaesthetic agent. These preparations survived for several hours.

b/ Experiments on chicks after hatching
These experiments were carried out on chicks from the time of hatching upto the adulthood. The heart rate of the animals was monitored from the pulse waves of the blood pressure measured electronically after cannulation of common carotid artery.
In this type of experiments the chicks were pretreated with pentobarbitone Na /Nembutal^R/ /100 mg/kg i.v./.

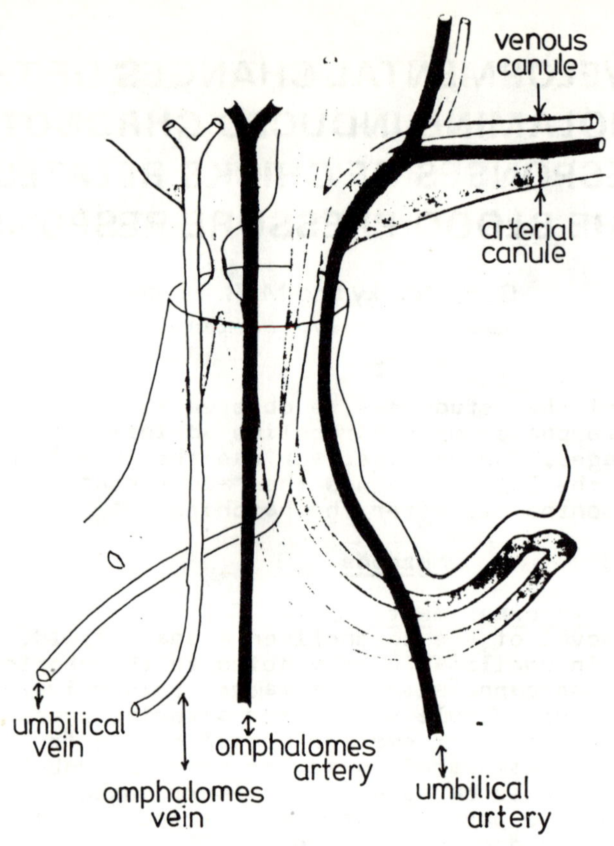

Fig. 1.: Schematic demonstration of the vessels at the umbilical region of the chick embryo. Upper part of the figure: extraembryonal vessels; below: intra-embryonal vessels. The arrows indicate the place of canule insertion.

Results

On the 11th incubational day, 1 ng/embryo dose of adrenaline provoked pressor response on blood pressure accompanied by tachycardia /Fig. 2./.

On the 13th embryonal day the reflex bradycardia did appeared within the adrenaline effect, but this heart rate response proved to be partly irreversible: it could not return to the initial level /Fig. 3./.

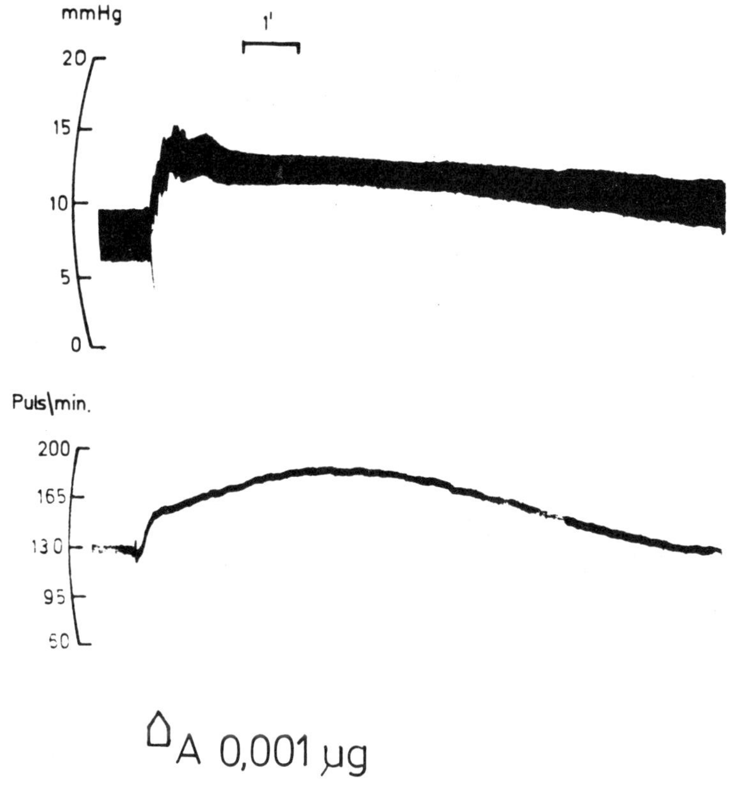

Fig. 2.: Blood pressure /upper row/ and heart rate
/bottom row/ responses of a chick embryo on the 11th
incubational day after adrenaline injection.

At the 17th embryonal day the reflex bradycardia became
evidently complete: the pulse rate also returned to a
nearly normal level after normalization of blood pressure
change /Fig. 4./.

The next figure /Fig. 5./ is to demonstrate the heart rate
responses of increasing adrenaline doses /0,25-16,0 ,ug/kg
i.v./ during several days of the first postembryonal/week
and on the following weeks upto the end of the 3rd posthatching month and lastly in adult hen.

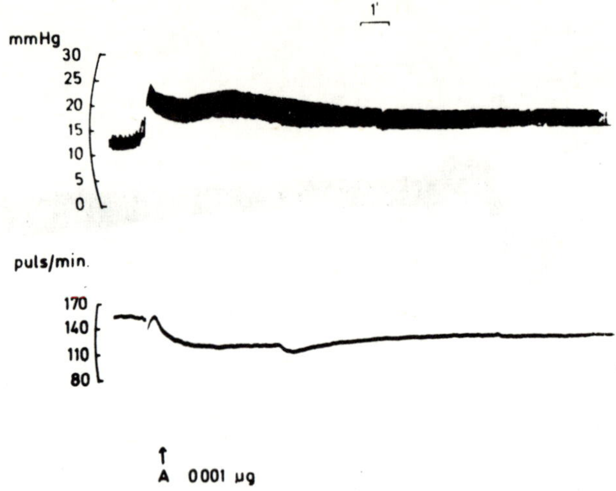

Fig. 3.: Blood pressure and heart rate responses of a chick embryo on the 13th incubational day after adrenaline injection.

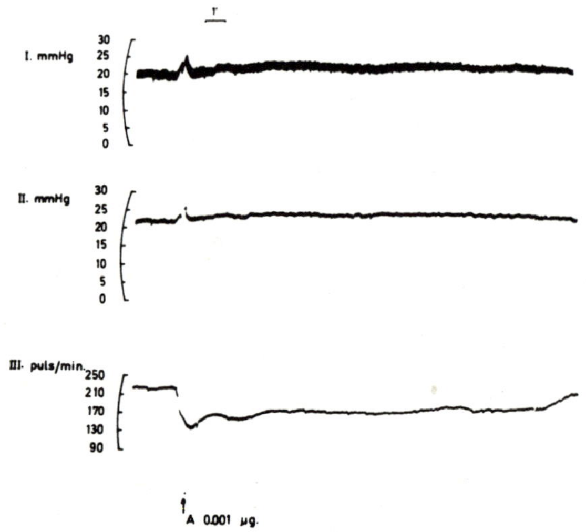

Fig. 4.: Blood pressure and heart rate responses of a 17th day old chick embryo upon adrenaline administration. Upper row: systemic pulsatile arterial pressure; bottom row: heart rate.

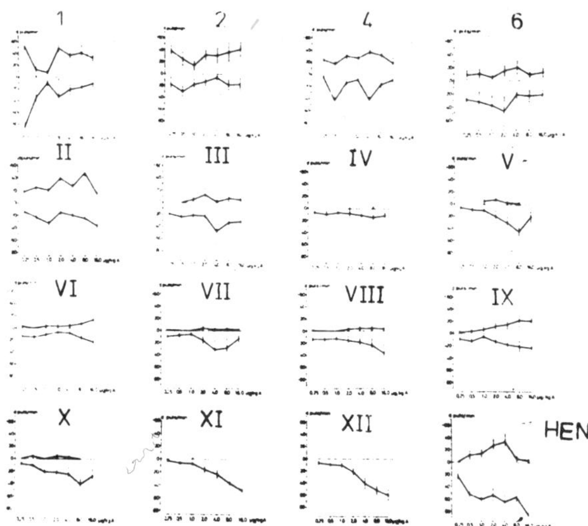

Fig. 5.: Heart rate responses of hatched chicks of
different ages upon increasing adrenaline doses
/0,25; 0,5; 1,0; 2,0; 4,0; 8,0 and 16,0 ug/kg i.v./.
First line: heart rate responses during the first
week after hatching /the days signed by arabic num-
bers/. Following lines: heart rate responses at several weeks after hatching and in case of "adult" hen
/i.e.: more than 3 months old/.
/Weeks are signed by Roman number/.

Just after the hatching, the heart rate responses proved to
be rather diverse: tachycardia and bradycardia equally
occured; the largest bradycardia appeared even after the
smallest dose. At the end of the first month, the heart rate
effect of adrenaline became transiently very weak, but,
thereafter, the reflex bradycardia gradually became more and
more prononuced and dose-dependent in height.

Discussion and Summary

By means of blood pressure measurement both in chick embryos
and chicks the chronotropic effects of adrenaline administrations could be detected along with the development of the
avian cardiovascular regulatory mechanism.
Although, at the mid-time of incubation the vegetative innervation of the cardiovascular system became nearly complete, its reflex regulation did not function.

In a 11th old chick embryo the reflex bradycardia in consequence of blood pressure elevation did not appear. Already,
before the hatching this cardio-inhibitory reflex went into
motion. However, during the "perinatal" period this reflex-
ogenic response seemed to be all-or-none type.

Only after the end of the first posthatching month became
the magnitude of reflex bradycardia dose-dependent and this
type of heart rate response upon adrenaline administration
proved to be characteristic for the later period of avian
life.

Discussion

Szentiványi: In previous studies performed many years ago by
my co-workers and myself /Szentiványi et al.: An ontogenetic
study of intracardiac ganglia. Acta physiol. Acad. Sci. hung.
21: 181-194, 1962/ we found that whereas the storage of myocardial catecholamines appears well developed at the date of
birth, or even before that date, the maturation of intracardiac sympathetic ganglia has a different time course: they do
not function until the tenth postnatal day. These studies were
carried out on embryonic and new-born rats. Could you relate,
perhaps, your very interesting results to some aspects of our
studies e.g. to the intriguingly protracted time course in
postnatal maturation of important cardiac adrenergic mechanism?

Rabloczky: Yes, in a sense, I can see some parallelism. The
extent or even the character of drug actions is modified in
chickens after hatching. There is a great sensitivity in chickens to vasodilator agents during the embryonic age. Isoproterenol e.g. could induce lethal hypotension. Later on, this
enormous sensitivity disappears. Interestingly enough, in the
case of anticholinesterases a total reversal of the blood pressure response was observed during the first 3 months after
hatching.
Some, but probably not all, of these changes are associated
with the fact that the blood-brain barrier becomes complete
for these agents.

Juhász-Nagy: We found that some agents of hypothalamic origin
such as vasopressin markedly dilate the avian coronaries.
Could you explain, as an expert of avian cardiovascular pharmacology, this strange discrepancy between mammals and birds?
Have you evidence of this difference?

Rabloczky: Yes, it is so. Vasopressin and related substances
not only dilate coronary vessels which are constricted in mammals on administration of these agents, but elicit a decrease
of systemic blood pressure, This is a species-dependent action
of the above substances, but, as far as I know, there is no
exact explanation for this fact.

THE PERIPHERAL INNERVATION
OF THE SMALL CORONARY VESSELS

M. Szentiványi, W. C. Randall, J. B. Pace and J. S. Wechsler
*Department of Physiology Loyala University, Stritch School of Medicine and the Graduate School
Hines, Illinois, USA*

In previous studies, nerve fibers coursing in the main branches
of the cardiac rami having a specific innervation to the coronary
vessels could be functionally separated from homologous fibers having
an augmentor action on myocardial contractility (Szentiványi and Kiss,
1957; Szentiványi and Juhász-Nagy, 1959; Szentiványi and Juhász-Nagy,
1961), and evidence was presented to indicate the former was represented at least in part by preganglionic fibers with synapses in or near
the heart. It has also been demonstrated that the nervous supply to
contractile elements of myocardium may be subdivided into small segments or units, thus permitting functional patterns of cardiac muscle
contraction (Szentiványi et al., 1967). Considering the very close
working relationship between the two systems (Szentiványi and Juhász-
Nagy, 1963a and 1963b; Juhász-Nagy et al. 1965; Belloni 1979), it
was reasonable to assume that the coronary innervation might also be
characterized by spatially restricted or localized responses. Thus, the
question was raised: does the coronary tree respond uniformly to
sympathetic nerve stimulation or can different portions of this tree be
separately excited as independent innervation units?

The purpose of this study was to evaluate the directional changes
in blood flow through discrete areas of the myocardium during separate
stimulation of cardiac nerve branches.

Methods
=======

Forty seven experiments were carried out on mongrel dogs (12-

20 kg) of either sex, under phencyclidine HCL (2 mg/kg) and chloralose (80 mg/kg) anesthesia. A modified heat clearance technique was employed in which two thermistors were used to assess changes of coronary blood flow in a given area. One thermistor was unheated and measured the actual temperature in the area, which served as reference for a second thermistor heated 1 $^{\circ}$C higher than the reference thermistor. The temperature recorded by the heated thermistor represents the algebraic sum of tissue heat and heat produced by passing a constant current through a high resistance element positioned in the needle tip. Hence, the temperature of the tissue locus heated by this thermistor depended upon the rate of blood flow perfusing the tissue (convective heat loss) as well as the metabolic heat production of the tissue. Since the reference thermistor measured tissue heat, the difference in temperature between it and the heated thermistor represented temperature fluctuations in the myocardium induced primarily by alterations in blood flow. The magnitude of flow change was expressed in percent by establishing the 0 flow value during a period of asystole and low perfusion pressure induced by strong vagal stimulation, the 100% value being the difference between 0 and control flow levels. The heated and reference thermistors were 1-2 mm apart and each inserted an equal distance (0. 5 - 1. 5 cm) into the left ventricular myocardium. To ascertain that both lay in a functionally homogenous area, vagal stimulation or adrenalin administration was carried out while both thermistors were unheated. If the thermistors were in proper position, the derived temperature differential equalled "0". Coronary constriction was indicated when the difference in temperature between the heated and unheated probes showed an increase above control values. On the other hand coronary dilation or increases in myocardial blood flow were signaled by a reduction in the temperature difference between the heated and unheated thermistors. The thermistor (2000 omega, Veco 32-A-7) and its heating wire were placed in a 20-21 gauge needle with a length of 3 - 3. 5 cm. These probes were so light that they were able to move with the heart without disturbance in position or recording stability.

In 15 experiments, coronary sinus flow was measured with a Morawitz cannula leading to an extracorporeal flow probe and electromagnetic flowmeter (Carolina Medical Electronics, Model 321). The sinus blood was returned to the right jugular vein. In these experiments 600 mg/kg heparin was administered. Spontaneous changes in sinus flow were generally paralleled by the local flow tracings, thus demonstrating the reliability of the thermistor method. Blood pressure was recorded from the right carotid by means of a Statham gauge, and was recorded together with force (Walton Brody Strain Gauge Arches) and flow tracings on a Grass polygraph. Branches of the stellate ganglia, as well as those from the caudal cervical ganglia, were carefully dissected free and stimulated at parameters of 5/sec, 4 msec and 8V.

Results

I. Coronary Constrictor Fibers. Table shows that vasoconstrictor responses to cardiac nerve stimulation were more frequently observed in local myocardial flow responses than in simultaneous recordings to coronary sinus outflow. Further, it is clear that peripheral sympathetic brances may contain a predominence of vasomotor fibers, whereas the main stellate branches may include a preponderance of chronotropic and inotropic fibers. In five experiments in which only the main branches of the stellate ganglia were stimulated, no constrictor responses were revealed by the recordings of total coronary sinus flow alone. The percentage of experiments in which constrictor response was elicited was increased by stimulating more peripheral sympathetic nerves while recording local flow changes by means of thermistor flow probes. Under these circumstances, coronary vasoconstriction was elicited in all 15 experiments (Table).

a) Figure 1 illustrates the variability in myocardial blood flow recorded from different regions of the left ventricle during stimulation of a small branch of the cardiac nerves.

Method of flow recroding	Ansa stimulation		Stimulation of peripherial branches		Number of exp.
	Constriction		Constriction		
	Yes	No	Yes	No	
Coronary sinus flow (flowmeter)	0	5	3	2	10
Local flow (thermistor)	8	8	15	0	31

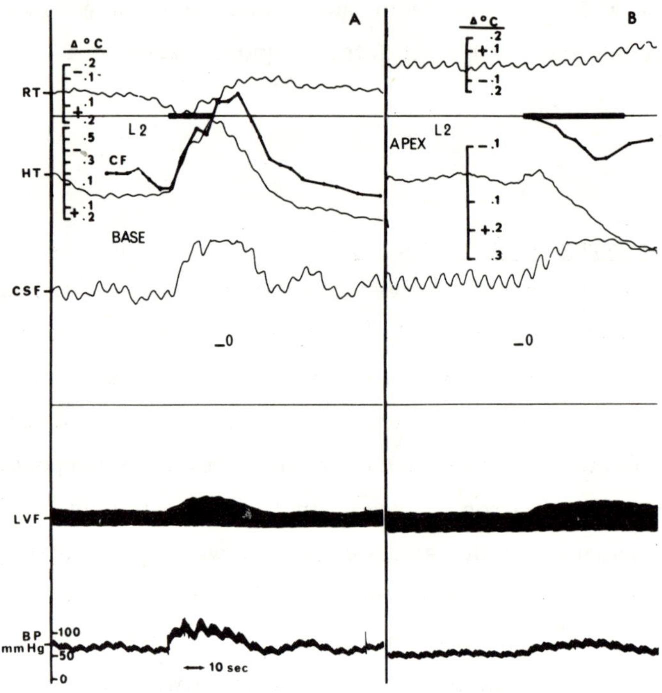

Fig. 1. Localized coronary constrictor response.
A) Left posterior ansa (L$_2$) stimulation caused metabolic dilatation at left ventricular base. Note how local flow and coronary sinus flow change in parallel manner.
B) The same nerve supplies the left ventricular apex with coronary constrictor fibers.
RT Reference (unheated thermistor, HT Heated thermistor, CF Local coronary flow as derived from HT (Heated thermistor) - RT (reference thermistor) values, CSF Coronary sinus flow recorded by an electromagnetic flowmeter, LVF Left ventricular force recorded by strain gauge, BP Blood pressure.

Stimulation of the left posterior ansa (L2) caused an elevation in blood pressure with both positive inotropic and chronotropic effects; coronary sinus flow (CSF) increased in association with increased cardiac vigor. Local flow in the myocardium of the LV base (CF) increased in parallel with overall flow (Figure 1A). However, local flow recorded from apical myocardium showed a sharp decrease even though coronary sinus flow increased (B), thus revealing a different distribution of vasoconstrictor fibers in this nerve.

In another instance, a large nerve carried metabolic dilator fibers while another, constrictor fibers to the same location. In figure 2A, local flow was measured in the left ventricular apex.

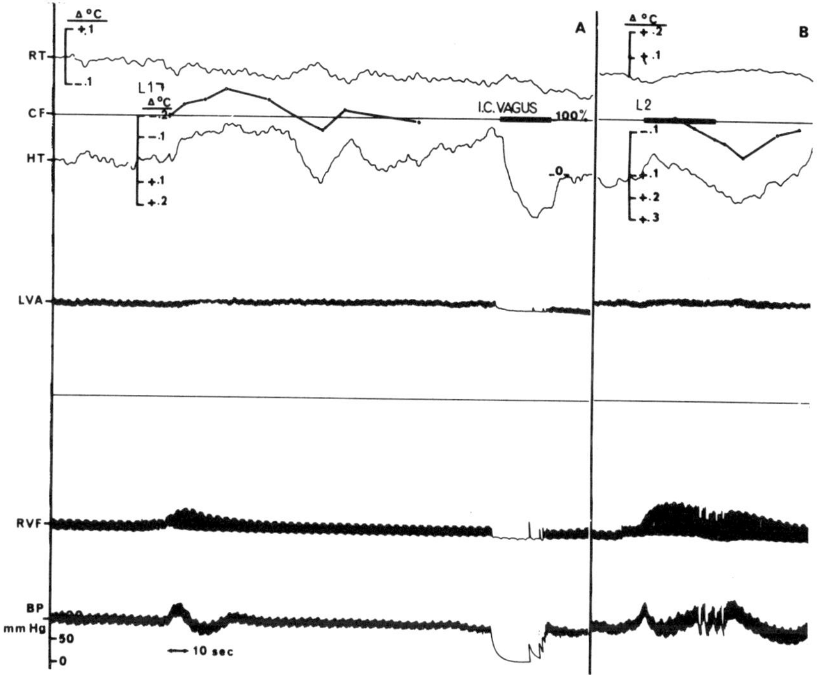

Fig. 2. Localized coronary constrictor response.
A) Left anterior ansa stimulation elicited a metabolic dilatation at left ventricular apex probes. Vagal stimulation to establish "0" flow. B) Posterior ansa stimulation caused a 70% decrease in CBF in the same location.
LVA Left ventricular apex force recorded by a strain gauge, RVF Right ventricular force, other symbols as in Fig. 1.

Stimulation of the left anterior ansa (L_1) caused an increased flow (CF), although the force of contraction of adjacent apical myocardium (LVA) was not changed. Thus, the flow increase was possibly related to increased perfusion pressure and/or increased metabolism which was not reflected in contractile force. On the other hand, when stimulating the posterior ansa L_2 (Figure 2B), the presence of constrictor fibers was manifest in a marked decrease in flow. Estimation of the range of control flow as compared with that during vagal stimulation revealed the decrease in flow was approximately 70% that of control values.

b) Figure 3A and 3B demonstrates how vasoconstrictor responses to cardiac nerve stimulation may not develop due to the profound metabolic responses resulting from stimulation of myocardial augmentor fibers. Electrical stimulation of branch (L_1) caused a great flow increase (Figure 3A). An equally pronounced decrease was elicited by stimulation of a peripheral branch (L_4) of the same nerve (Figure 3B). The administration of hexamethonium abolished the constrictor effects of L4 stimulation, however, the metabolic dilation resulting from L1 stimulation was still evident.

c) Another way to unmask coronary constrictor response is to deprive a large nerve of its dilator branches, thus isolating the vasoconstrictor fibers. In figure 4, left anterior ansa stimulation induced only a comparatively small flow increase (A), suggesting that concurrent stimulation of both constrictor and metabolic dilator fibers may damp the flow change. Actually, L_5, a branch of the sympathetics (B), or the thoracic trunk of the degenerated vagus (C) descending from the caudal cervical ganglion caused a relatively large flow increase, while myocardial force remained relatively unaffected (B, C). These results indicated that these nerves did not contain many constrictor fibers. After transecting these two potent dilator components, the constrictor elements of the anterior ansa (L1) then elicited relatively unopposed action (D, E).

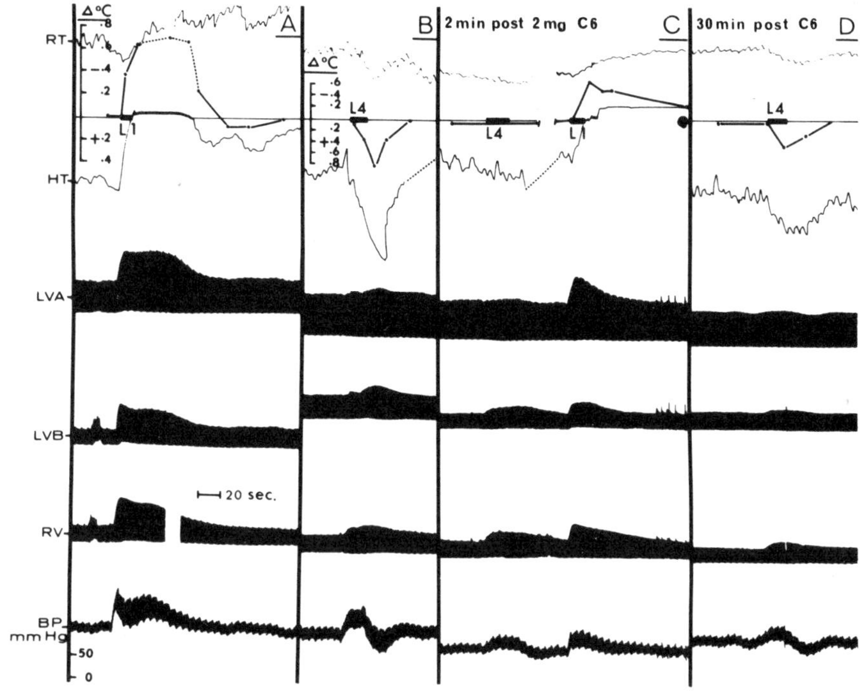

Fig. 3. Coronary constrictor effect of a peripheral branch of the left stellate due to the presence of preganglionic vasomotor fibers.
A) Left anterior ansa (L_1) stimulation elicited a strong metabolic dilation in the left ventricular apex segment.
B) L_4, one of the peripheral branches of L_1, contained constrictor fibers.
C) 2 mg of hexamethonium (C_6) administered into the coronary artery perfusing the area where flow was measured blocked constriction without interfering with metabolic dilatation and cardiac action of L_1 and L_4.
D) After the elimination of C_6, the constrictor response of L_4 reappears.
LVA Left ventricular apex, LVB Left ventricular base, RV Right ventricle.
Force of contraction measured by strain gauge arches.
Other symbols as in figure 1.

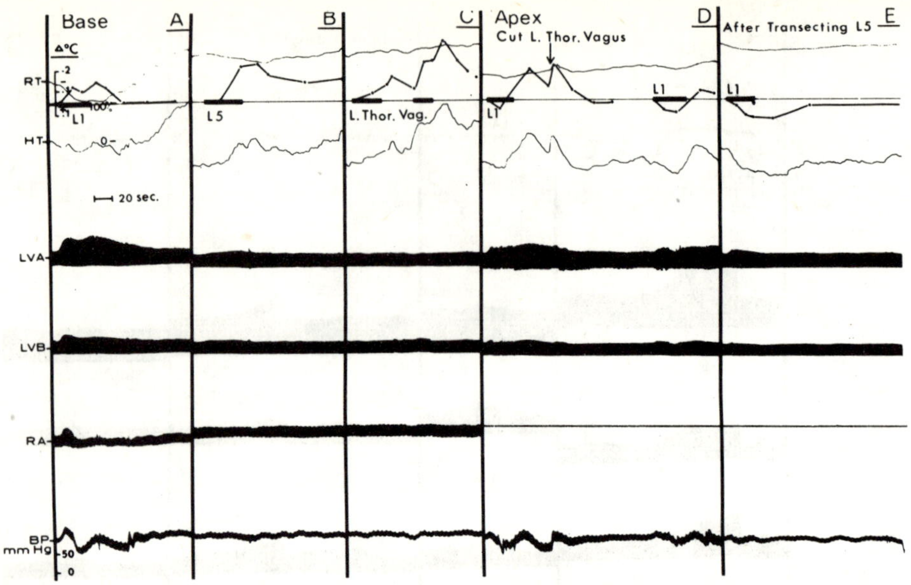

Fig. 4. The resulting coronary constrictor response of a main sympathetic branch after transecting its dilator branches.
A) Left anterior ansa (L_1) acts as a metabolic dilator nerve at left ventricular base.
B) L_5, a branch of L_1, caused considerable dilator response.
C) The degenerated left thoracic vagus is similarly a very potent dilator at left ventricular apex. (Vagus was cut in the neck, rostral to the caudal cervical ganglion 16 days before the experiment.)
D) After transecting the left thoracic vagus, L_1 has a preliminary flow decreasing effect, besides its dilator action, suggesting that this nerve also contains constrictor fibers to this area. After cutting one of its dilator branches, this constrictor response increased.
E) After transecting L_5, the stimulation of L_1 decreased flow by 50% (The stimulation was performed after atropinization (0.32 mg/kg).
Symbols as in figures 1 and 2.

II. The Peripheral Course of Vasoconstrictor Fibers. In seven experiments, by carefully stripping the epicardium from different portions of the heart surface, and by cleaning the left common coronary artery and its anterior descending branch, an attempt was made to define the peripheral course of the vasomotor fibers and their relationship to contractile myocardial fiber pathways. Changes in local flow and myocardial contractions were observed before and after these procedures. As a main result, constrictor responses which were generally masked before localized denervation became more and more visible as epicardial denervation progressed. Epicardial stripping, which extinguished most contractile responses to both left and right ansa stimulation, did not alter the constrictor effects, especially when the right sympathetics were stimulated. Thus, vasomotor fibers from the right stellate to the left ventricular apex may avoid routes used by contractile fibers and reach the region through other channels, possibly via right coronary pathways. When the major part of the posterior cardiac plexus was removed, leaving intact only its most lateral portion, right sympathetic stimulation caused only a mechanical effect on the right atrium and a vasoconstrictor response on the left ventricular apex.

III. The Coronary Nerves. Figure 5 illustrates the response to stimulation of sympathetic brances found in the region of the left common coronary artery in 12 experiments. Stimulation of a large branch of a nerve trunk penetrating the artery (N. Cor.) caused a very marked coronary constriction without change in contractile force or blood pressure (Figure 5B). Other nerves (C_1) which did not penetrate the coronary artery wall caused an increase of cardiac force with a concomitant augmentation in flow (5A). The schematic drawing (Figure 5C) reveals additional accessory fibers (broken lines) which penetrated the coronary arteries. Their stimulation also caused decreased myocardial perfusion around the thermistor probe.

IV. The Quality of the Constrictor Fibers. The local administration of drugs influencing the target area only proved useful in distinguishing between vasomotor and contractile fibers (Figure 3C).

Close arterial injection of hexamethonium (C_6) extinguished the constrictor response to simulation without interference with the mechanical effects. As the influence of this drug diminished vasomotor effects reappeared (Figure 3D).

The cardioaccelerator fibers contained in the peripheral branches of the ansae are thought to be primarily postganglionic, having their

relay stations in the stellate and caudal cervical ganglia. The vasomotor fibers appear to be primarily preganglionic (Szentiványi and
Kiss, 1957; Szentiványi and Juhász-Nagy, 1959).

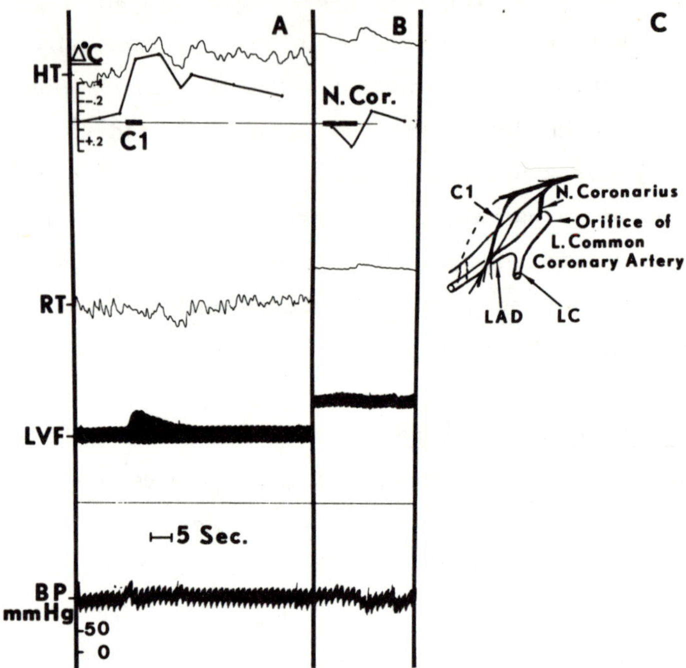

Fig. 5. The nervus coronarius.
A) Nerve C_1, which bypassed the region of the left common
coronary artery, elicited a contractile response.
B) A large branch which apparently penetrated the artery (n. coronarius) elicited a considerable flow decrease without any change
in the cardiac contractility.
C) Anatomical course of the fibers in the region of the left common
coronary artery.
LAD Left anterior descending artery, LC Left circumflex of the
left coronary artery.

In the experiment represented by figure 6, a large sympathetic
nerve distal to the left caudal cervical ganglion was stimulated. Excitation elicited a biphasic action, an initial contriction followed by
metabolic dilation (6A). By decreasing the stimulation voltage to 3V (B),
preganglionic vasomotor fibers were preferentially stimulated; this
stimulation elicited a 50% constriction without concomitant change in

36

muscle contractility and without a secondary increase in flow. Such
phenomena were observed in six experiments.

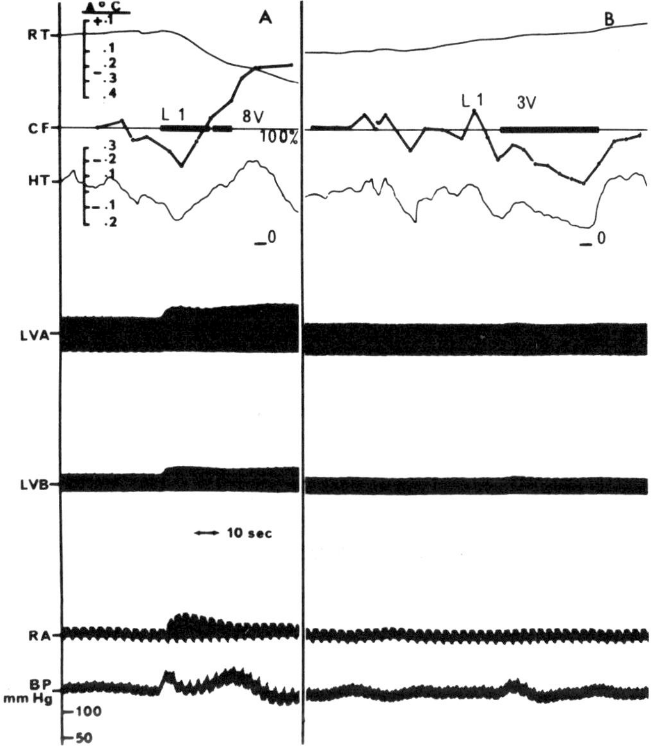

Fig. 6. Discrimination between vasomotor and myocardial fibers.
A) L_1 (large branch of left caudal cervical ganglion) stimulation
followed by a biphasic change in flow.
B) Stimulation with low intensity (3 volts) selectively revealed the
constrictor response. No change in cardiac force and no metabolic
dilation was present.
RA Right atrial contractile force measured by a strain gauge.
Other symbols as in figures 1 and 2.

V. The Dilator Fibers in the Autonomic Outflow to the Heart.

In the present experiments, the following types of dilator responses
were observed:

a) Flow increase associated with augmented cardiac contractility
not blocked by atropine.

b) A dilator response observed without concomitant changes in
cardiac force, and also not blocked by atropine, but presumably related to local metabolic changes.

37

c) Increase in flow, which could be blocked by atropine and which was not accompanied by changes in cardiac contractility. Figure 7 illustrates such a case.

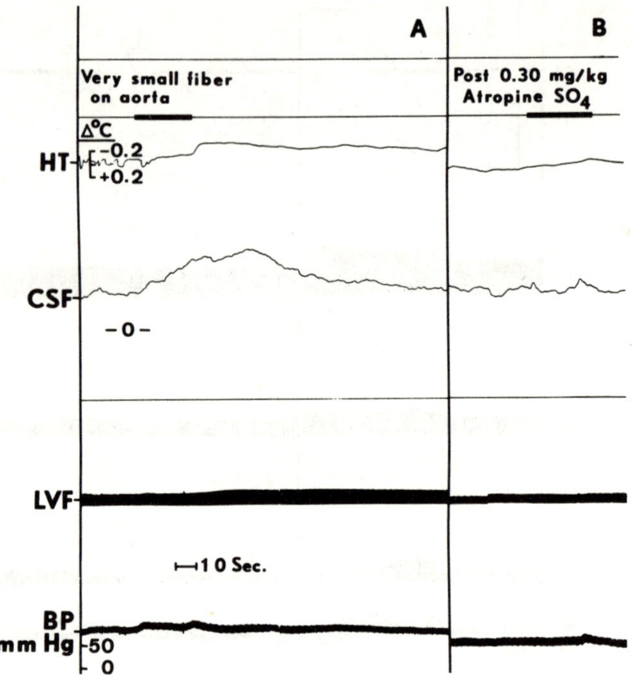

Fig. 7. Peripheral sympathetic cholinergic dilator fiber.
A) Dilation measured locally by a heated thermistor (HT) and an electromagnetic flowmeter from coronary sinus (CSF)
B) Atropine blocked the dilatatation.
Other symbols as in figures 1 and 2.

Stimulation of a fine branch of the aortic plexus elicited a flow increase as recorded locally by the heated thermistor and from the coronary sinus by means of an electromagnetic flowmeter (7A). The stimulation did not change the myocardial contractile force of the test segment. Atropine blocked this dilator effect (7B).

Discussion

An important new observation in these experiments focuses upon the localized nature of vasomotor innervation and response. The coronary tree appears to consist of separate and independent innervation

38

units, a concept which corresponds well with that has been described for the neural control of the contractile myocardium (Szentiványi et al., 1967). It is therefore evident that different portions of the ventricle (base and apex in the present experiments) are supplied by different portions of the cardiac sympathetic nerves. However, there is good reason to believe that individual vessel segments are also supplied by nerves which overlap with those going to adjacent contractile myocardium.

Stimulation of a fiber which failed to produce vasoconstriction in a given area was frequently found to be effective when the thermistor probes were moved just a few millimeters distance. Similarly a close relationship between myocardial augmentor and coronary constrictor fibers were found in the hypothalamic representation of the two systems (Juhász-Nagy et al., 1965). Perhaps these results explain the failure of some workers to elicit a clear constrictor response to sympathetic stimulation. However, Berne et al. (1965), as well as (Granata et al., 1965), found a shortlasting flow decrease which preceded metabolic dilator effects, concluding that it might be due to constrictor fiber stimulation.

It may rightly be assumed that coronary vasoconstrictor responses compete with metabolic vasodilation even during periods of the preponderance of the latter. The validity of this assumption, held formerly untenable by most workers in this field, has recently been shown by Mohrman and Feigl (1978). These authors estimated from their results that alpha-adrenoceptor mediated vasoconstriction attenuates, by approximately 30 percent, the coronary flow increase induced by adrenergic excitation or carotid hypotension. Subsequently, a latent vasoconstrictor influence was also shown to attenuate the decrease of coronary vascular resistance during periods of high sympathetic discharge as occurs during exercise in the conscious dog (Murray and Vatner, 1979). Moreover, the sympathetic nervous system appears to exert a tonic constrictor effect on the coronary vessels: stellate ganglion ablation (Schwartz and Stone, 1977) or administration of alpha-blocking agents (Aviado and Juhász-Nagy, this symposium) result in an increased myocardial perfusion under stressful conditions. Unmasking the coronary vasoconstrictor effect by beta-antagonists is also a well established fact. However, the above - cited works permitted the analysis of the presence and magnitude of the coronary vasoconstrictor effects only by an indirect way. Workers have failed to induce coronary vasoconstriction directly while stimulating the stellate or its main branches and measuring flow in large vessels in animals untreated with beta-blocking agents. The present experiments were also generally unable to show convincing constrictor changes in these large vascular channels. However, when peripheral stimulation was combined with local, small vessel bed flow measurements, there was no experiment in which coronary constriction could not be observed. Masking metabolic dilator effects were avoided by isolating and stimulating branches which contained mainly constrictor fibers. Since such constrictor responses were often restricted to a small circumscribed area of the myocardium, this effect would not be manifest in the face of simultaneous metabolic dilation involving more extensive areas of the left ventricle. The magnitude of flow decrease measured by local thermistor probes thus represented local changes without involving unknown changes in flow at distant areas. Local flow generally changed from 30 to 50%, and not infrequently a 70% decrease was observed. These values indicate a potentially important constrictor innervation, which may play a prominent role in the regulation of coronary blood distribution and flow.

The effect of peripheral stimulation with local tissue flow measurement provides an excellent opportunity to study the nature of the constrictor fibers. Earlier studies have demonstrated that branches divided from the stellate ganglion of the cat contain preganglionic B fibers which supply the coronaries (Szentiványi and Kiss, 1957; Szentiványi and Juhász-Nagy, 1959) and which form synapses in intra-cardiac ganglia. Preganglionic B fibers could be selectively activated with low voltage stimulation and functionally separated from post ganglionic C fibers innervating the myocardium. In dogs (Juhász-Nagy and

40

Szentiványi, 1961), this separation is not easy at the level of the main
stellate branches, owing to the fact that many myocardial fibers are
also preganglionic at this level, and make synapses in the caudal cervical ganglion. During stimulation of peripheral branches distal to the
latter ganglion, the separation was easier since myocardial fibers are
postganglionic while the vasomotor fibers are preganglionic. Accordingly, in the present studies, lowering the stimulation voltage regularly
caused constriction, whithout obvious changes in values of cardiac
performance, provided the stimulated branch contained appropriate constrictor fibers.

Similar conclusions may be drawn from blocking the intracardiac
ganglia by Hexamethonium (C_6). Local administration of C_6 in small
doses produced, without side effects, reversible blockade of vasoconstrictor responses to nerve stimulation. Such experiments produced convincing confirmation of the presence of ganglionic cell stations which
mediated vasomotor changes in the myocardium.

Although the coronary constrictor fibers may supply the same
segments as the myocardial fibers, they do not necessarily follow the
same course. Denervations which abolish the myocardial response may
even amplify a local constrictor response.

The precise distribution of the constrictor fibers was not followed
in these experiments although it seems clear that at least some such
fibers may course from the right stellate to the left ventricular apex
via the right coronary plexus. It is also probable that most of the constrictor fibers run in the coronary plexus. Thus, the right stellate,
which has a considerable compartment of fibers projecting to the epicardial plexus, may lose its myocardial contractile effect as a result
of epicardial ablations, without loss of its vasoconstrictor action.

Nerve branches of considerable size were found in the region of
the left common coronary artery, some of which penetrated the artery
wall. Stimulation of these nerves caused pronounced flow decreases
without generalized changes in cardiac contractile force. The anatomical course of these branches showed considerable variation, but two

main patterns emerged. In most animals, a large nerve coursed
parallel to the common coronary, either closely adjacent to the vessel
or in the accompanying fat pad. When a large branch penetrated per-
pendicularly into the left common coronary or the origin of one of its
branches, it was designated the nervus coronarius. Its electrical stimulation regularly produced strong diminution in flow. In some
animals, a parallel branch emitted a number of small perpendicular
branches to the common or LAD, which were called nervi coronarii
accessorii.

Summary

In 47 experiments, local myocardial blood flow was measured by
means of paired thermistors, placed 1 to 2 mm apart, with one heated
to a temperature 1 $^{\circ}$C higher than the other which recorded true,
local tissue temperature. Coronary sinus outflow was measured simultaneously. The largest, as well as the smallest branches of the cardiac sympathetic nerves were electrically stimulated. Coronary vasoconstrictor nerves separately innervate different segments of the coronary tree. Although the areas innervated by the coronary system
may coincide with those of the contractile myocardium, the course
of the vasomotor fibers appears to be different from that which medi-
ates changes in contractile force.

In the left common coronary region, nerve branches were described which penetrate the vessel and when stimulated, elicit a strong
vasoconstrictor response. The coronary vasomotor fibers appear to
be preganglionic; their threshold for excitation is lower than that of
the postganglionic myocardial contractile fibers. Close arterial injection of C_6 abolishes the localized constrictor response. A close relationship between cardiac metabolic fibers and the coronary constrictor systems is indicated.

42

References

Belloni, F. L.: The local control of coronary blood flow.
  Cardiovasc. Res. 13: 63-85, 1979
Berne, R. M., deGeest, H. and Levy, M.: Influence of the cardiac
  nerves on coronary resistance. Am. J. Physiol. 208: 763-769,
  1965
Granata, L., Olsson, R.A., Huvos, A., and Gregg, D.E.: Coronary
  inflow and oxygen usage following cardiac sympathetic nerve stimu-
  lation in unanesthetized dogs. Circ. Res. 16: 114-120, 1965
Juhász-Nagy, A., Szentiványi, M.: Separation of cardioaccelerator and
  coronary vasomotor fibers in the dog. Am. J. Physiol. 200:
  125-129, 1961
Juhász-Nagy, A., Szentiványi, M., Ovary, I. and Debreczeni, L.:
  Hypothalamic control of coronary circulation in the dog. Arch.
  Internat. de Physiol. et de Biochimie, 73: 798-816, 1965
Mohrman, D.E., and Feigl, E.O.: Competition between sympathetic
  vasoconstriction and metabolic vasodilation in the canine coronary
  circulation. Circ. Res. 42: 79-86, 1978
Murray, P.A. and Vatner, S.E.: Alpha-adrenoceptor attenuation of
  the coronary vascular response to severe exercise in the conscious
  dog. Circ. Res. 45: 654-660, 1979
Randall, W.C., Szentiványi, M., Pace, J.B., Wechsler, J.S.,
  Kaye, M.P.: Patterns of sympathetic nerve projections onto the
  canine heart. Circ. Res. 22: 315-323, 1968
Schwartz, P.J. and Stone, H.L.: Tonic influence of the sympathetic
  nervous system on myocardial reactive hyperemia and on coronary
  blood flow distribution. Circ. Res. 41: 51-58, 1977
Szentiványi, M. and Juhász-Nagy, A.: A new aspect of the nervous
  control of the coronary blood vessels. Quart. J. Exper. Physiol.
  44: 67-79, 1959
Szentiványi, M. and Juhász-Nagy, A.: The physiological role of the
  coronary constrictor fibres. I. The effect of the coronary vasomotors on the systemic blood pressure. Quart. J. Exper. Physiol.
  48: 93-104, 1963a
Szentiványi, M. and Juhász-Nagy, A.: The physiological role of the
  coronary constrictor fibres. II. The role of coronary vasomotors
  in metabolic adaptation of the coronaries. Quart. J. Exper. Physiol.
  48: 105-118, 1963b
Szentiványi, M. and Kiss, E.: Beitrage zur Innervation der Koronar-
  gefaesse, Acta Physiol. Acad. Sci. Hung. 11: 347-356, 1957.
Szentiványi, M., Pace, J.B., Wechsler, J.S., and Randall, W.C.:
  Localized myocardial responses to stimulation of cardiac sympathetic nerves. Circ. Res. 21: 691-702, 1967.

INVERSE RECIPROCAL REGULATION OF CARDIAC POST-SYNAPTIC α- AND β- ADRENOCEPTORS BY THYROID HORMONES

George Kunos

Department of Pharmacology, McGill University, 3655 Drummond Street, Montreal, Quebec H3G 1Y6
Canada

The study of adrenergic receptors has been one of the most active research fields in modern pharmacology. Paradoxically, the first suggestion of the existence of different kinds of adrenergic receptors by Henry Dale was on a physiological basis, to explain the antagonistic effects of adrenaline in different, or, sometimes, in the same tissue. Later, Ahlquist (1948) classified adrenergic receptors pharmacologically, on the basis of different potency orders for agonists. As Ahlquist's classification has become widely accepted, it has also become obvious that in some tissues the same biological end response can be mediated by either basic type – α or β – receptor. This apparent redundancy on the part of nature may have survival values: α and β adrenergic receptors usually activate different biochemical pathways with different metabolic consequences, and a change in their relative contribution to the final tissue response may serve to adapt tissue function to metabolic state. The first suggestion that the relative dominance of α- and β-receptors may be governed by the metabolic state of the tissue came from a study of isolated frog hearts. Kunos and Szentivanyi (1968) reported that the inotropic effect of adrenaline was preferentially inhibited by a β-receptor antagonist at higher and by an α-receptor antagonist at lower temperatures. It was also found that irreversible block of α-receptors by phenoxybenzamine at a low temperature prevented the appearance of β-receptors when the temperature of the same preparation was raised (Kunos & Nickerson, 1976). We proposed that a single basic type of adrenergic receptor, whose properties – α or β – change with temperature could explain this observation. Our findings were confirmed by several laboratories using spontaneously beating amphibian heart preparations. In electrically driven preparations, where complications may arise by autonomic transmitter release and its enhancement at low temperatures, some workers failed to detect reciprocal changes in α- and β-responses, while others did detect such a shift but in a direction opposite to that found in spontaneously beating preparations. Temperature-alteration of cardiac α and β-receptor responses has been recently discussed elsewhere (Nickerson & Kunos, 1977; Kunos, 1978, 1980; Kunos & Preiksaitis, 1978), and in this paper some of our observations on the modulation of cardiac adrenoceptors by thyroid hormones are presented.

Thyroid dysfunction has long been known to influence the sympathetic reactivity of the myocardium, but the mechanism of this interaction was obscure. Even before the advent of ligand binding techniques, two developments gave new impetus to research in this area. The first was the

realization that positive inotropic and chronotropic responses to sympa-
thomimetics can be mediated by either β- or α-receptors in the heart, and
the second was the use of selective α- and β-adrenergic drugs that allowed
analysis of the relative contribution of the two receptors to the net
tissue response in different thyroid states.

In an organ where the same end response to a hormone is mediated by
two different receptors, some predictions can be made as to what type of
changes in drug effects are expected if the relative numbers of the two
receptors, in this case α and β, is altered. It is important to discuss
these briefly because many of the arguments recently raised against the
existence of such changes were based on erroneous assumptions. Firstly,
there should be a change in the relative potency of agonists with different
relative activities on α- and β-receptors. Secondly, there should be
changes in the effects of adrenoceptor antagonists, but only in certain
conditions. Interaction between a selective agonist and a selective antagonist of the same receptor (e.g. isoproterenol - propranolol) is only
determined by the affinity of the receptor to the antagonist and should
not be influenced by a change in the absolute or relative numbers of receptors. However, the degree of block of the effect of a mixed agonist by
a high concentration of a selective antagonist is determined by the number
or availability of the second type of receptor not susceptible to the
antagonist. If the latter is changed, the degree of apparent block will
change inversely. This relationship is illustrated by findings of Schu-
mann et al. (1974), whose results show that the Schild-plot for block of
the inotropic responses of the mixed α-β agonist phenylephrine by phentolamine is very flat, but the slope becomes steeper and close to the theoretical value of 1.0 in preparations preincubated with a β-receptor antagonist.

Hypothyroidism induced by thyroidectomy or hypophysectomy in rats
shifted the ratio of adrenoceptors from β to α, as suggested by findings
predicted above (Kunos, 1977; Kunos et al., 1980). In left atria of
hypophysectomized rats the potency of isoproterenol decreased and the
potency of the pure α-receptor agonist methoxamine increased (Fig. 1).
These changes developed slowly over 6-12 weeks, but they were rapidly and
completely reversed within 2 days by in vivo treatment of T4 that did not
cause significant cardiac hypertrophy. Hypothyroidism also reduced base-
line cardiac contractility and altered the efficacy of agonists, but these
changes were unaffected by the short T4 treatment. This indicates that
the latter changes were probably non-specific consequences of the cardiac
atrophy associated with prolonged hypothyroidism. In contrast to the
effects of T4, treatment of hypophysectomized rats with cortisone was
without any effect on the potency of agonists. The inhibitory potency of
propranolol against isoproterenol (Hashimoto & Nakashima, 1978) or of
phentolamine against methoxamine (Nakashima et al., 1973) in rat left
atria is not altered by hypothyroidism, indicating that the affinity of
cardiac β- and α-adrenoceptors, respectively, is unaltered by thyroid
hormones. However, as predicted for a change in receptor numbers, responses to the mixed agonist phenylephrine were blocked by α-receptor antagonists more effectively and by β-receptor antagonists less effectively
in hypothyroid than in euthyroid preparations (Fig. 2). Similarly, a
Schild-plot of the block of inotropic responses to noradrenaline by propranolol became flat with a slope of significantly less than 1.0 in hypothyroid left atria, indicating the appearance of an α-component in the
effect of this agonist (Kunos et al., 1980).

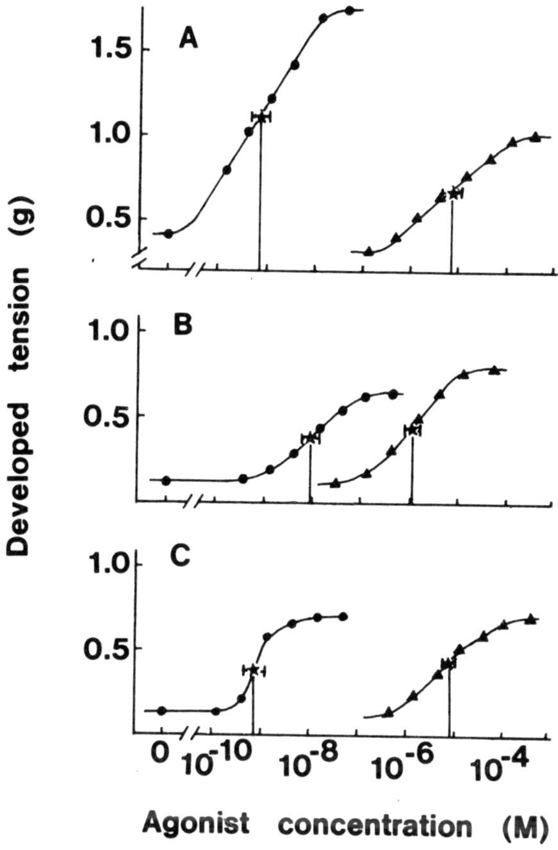

Fig. 1. Inotropic responses of left atria to isoprenaline (●) and to methoxamine (▲) in normal (a), hypophysectomized (b), and hypophysectomized rats treated for 2 days with thyroxine 0.2 mg/kg daily (c). Number of experiments: 4 (a); 4 (b); 3 (c). The asterisks on the dose-response curves and the horizontal bars indicate the mean EC_{50} ± 2 x s.e. The vertical lines were drawn to illustrate mean EC_{50}S on the abscissae. Reproduced by permission from Kunos et al. (1980).

These indirect indications of a change in the ratio of α- and β-receptors without changes in their affinities could be confirmed by ligand binding studies. There are a number of important considerations in the design of such experiments and the assessment of their results: 1. Binding sites should be determined in total tissue homogenate rather than purified membrane fragments because of the low and possibly uneven yield of receptors in the latter in different thyroid states; 2. Prolonged thyroid dysfunction is known to cause profound changes in membrane structure and composition. The best way to minimize errors that such changes may cause in the estimation of receptor densities is to compare hypothyroid preparations before and after a short-term thyroid hormone treatment; 3. The identity of 'specific' binding sites for radioligands with receptors mediating a well defined physiological function should be rigorously tested. For example,

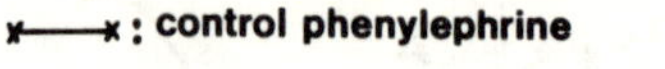

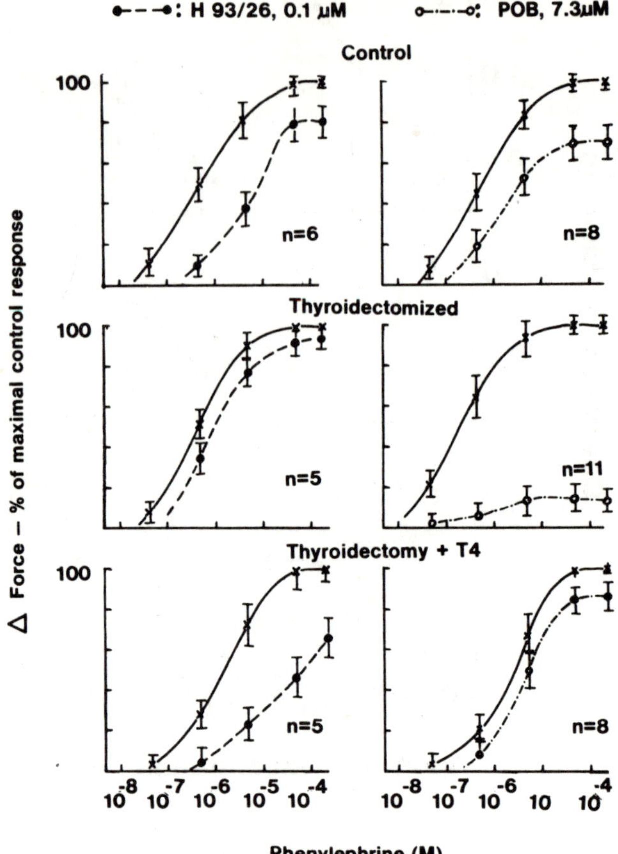

Fig. 2. The effect of thyroid state on the sensitivity of the inotropic effect of phenylephrine to α- and β-receptor blockade. Mean
phenylephrine dose response curves from electrically driven rat
left atria are shown x———x: control curves, ●－－●: in the presence
of 0.1 μM metoprolol (H93/26) o－·－o: after incubation with POB
(7.3 μM, 40 min.).

several recent studies indicate that ^{3}H-dihydroalprenolol (DHA) labels β-
receptors with high affinity ($K_d \leq 2$ nM), and propranolol suppressible
binding at ligand concentrations above 3-4 nM are largely non-specific
(Nahorski & Richardson, 1979; Winek & Bhalla, 1979). For α-receptors,
both the labeled and the suppressing ligand should preferably be α_1-
selective, to avoid labeling of presynaptic α-receptors. Dihydroergocryptine labels both α_1 and α_2 receptors, although α_1 receptors are preferentially labeled at ligand concentrations under 3 nM (Guicheney et al.,
1978; Kunos et al., 1979). When adrenoceptor binding sites were identified in ventricular homogenates from hypophysectomized rats and from
similar animals treated for 2 days with 0.2 mg/kg T_4, the density of high

affinity DHA binding sites increased, and there was a matching decrease in
the density of prazosin suppressible ^{3}H-WB-4101 binding sites (Kunos et
al., 1980). The latter two ligands are post-synaptic selective α-receptor
antagonists. The dissociation constant of DHA or WB-4101 remained unchanged and the affinity of the α-receptor binding site to methoxamine or
the β-receptor binding site to isoproterenol was also not affected by the
T_4 treatment (Fig. 3, Table 1). These findings indicate that thyroid-
dependent reciprocal changes in cardiac α- and β-receptor reactivity are
associated with and, probably, due to similar inverse, and matching,
changes in the density of postsynaptic α- and β-adrenoceptors.

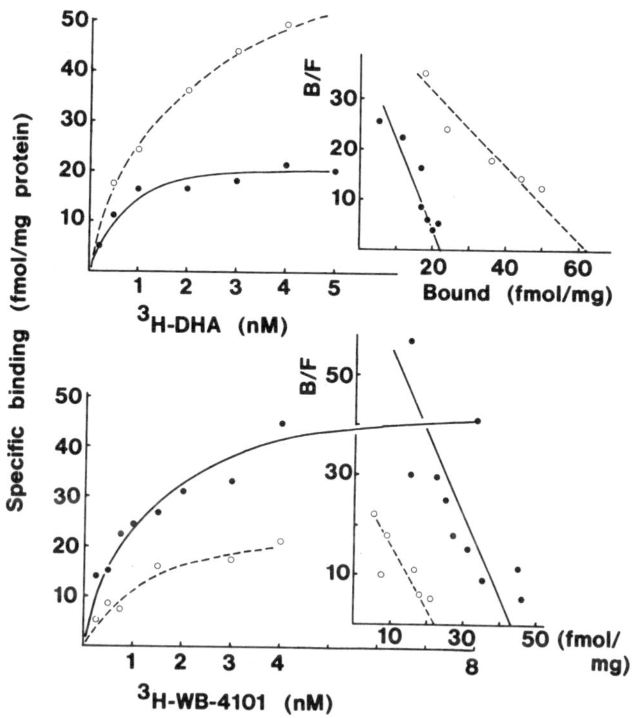

Fig. 3. The effect of thyroxine treatment of hypophysectomized rat
on the specific binding of ^{3}H -WB-4101 and ^{3}H -dihydroalprenolol
(^{3}H -DHA) to cardiac membrane fragments. ($\bullet$) Hypophysectomized
rat: (O) hypophysectomized rat treated with T4 0.2 mg/kg daily for
2 days. Insets are Scatchard-plots. Reproduced by permission from
Kunos et al. (1980).

Next, I will discuss some of our recent findings that indicate an
interesting interaction between thyroid hormones and sympathetic innervation in the regulation of postsynaptic cardiac adrenoceptors (Kunos et
al., 1980). The discovery of this interaction was fortuitous: we sympa-
thetically denervated hypothyroid rats to eliminate sites of neuronal uptake for noradrenaline. In normal hearts phenoxybenzamine potentiates the
effects of noradrenaline, an effect partly due to block of neuronal uptake.

Table 1. The effect of thyroxine treatment of hypophysectomized rats on the numbers and affinities of α_1 and β-adrenoceptor binding sites

| | ^{3}H-WB-4101 binding (α_1) | | | ^{3}H-DHA binding (β) | | | Total |
	Density (fmol/mg p.)	Affinity (K_d, nM)	K_d:methoxamine (μM)	Density	Affinity	K_d:isoprenaline (μM)	$\alpha_1 + \beta$
Hypophys-ectomized	38.7 $\pm$3.1 (4)	0.48 $\pm$0.08	6.5	27.5 $\pm$2.7 (6)	1.59 $\pm$0.27	0.45	66.2
Hypophys-ectomized + T$_4$	18.7** $\pm$2.5 (4)	0.60 $\pm$0.18	8.9	45.5* $\pm$5.7 (5)	1.89 $\pm$0.28	0.32	64.2

The K_d of methoxamine was determined at 2 nM ^{3}H-WB-4101, and the K_d of isoprenaline at 2 nM ^{3}H-DHA. Values shown are means from 2 separate experiments and are calculated as K_d = IC_{50}/[1+(2/K_d labelled ligand)]. Treatment with l-thyroxine was 0.2 mg/kg daily for 2 days. Asterisks indicate significant difference from corresponding value in untreated hypophysectomized rats; *P < 0.01; **P < 0.001. Number of experiments in parentheses. Binding site densities and affinities were obtained from Scatchard plots in individual experiments (5 to 8 points). Reproduced by permission from Kunos et al. (1980).

We argued that elimination of the neuronal uptake mechanism could unmask or potentiate the α-blocking effect of phenoxybenzamine in hypothyroid preparations. Unexpectedly, we found the opposite: denervation of hypothyroid rats by 6-hydroxydopamine (6-OHDA) potentiated responses to noradrenaline, but this effect was not inhibited at all by phenoxybenzamine, and even the block of effect of phenylephrine, an amine not substrate for uptake$_1$, was significantly reduced after denervation. This suggested that denervation may have prevented the shift in receptors caused by hypothyroidism, and this was confirmed in experiments with the β-receptor antagonist propranolol and with agonists. In denervated hypothyroid atria the blocking effect of propranolol against the mixed agonist noradrenaline was identical to its effect in denervated euthyroid atria, and the slope of Schild-plots was close to 1.0 in both cases. Thus, the flat slope observed in hypothyroid preparations was eliminated by denervation. The potency of agonists was also reversed: the potency of isoproterenol increased and the potency of phenylephrine decreased to levels seen in control atria, whereas the potency of noradrenaline increased beyond control values, due to denervation supersensitivity.

To determine whether the absence of normal stores of the neurotransmitter or of some other factors related to intact sympathetic innervation was responsible for the observed effects of denervation, we studied the responses of atria from hypothyroid rats treated with reserpine to deplete noradrenaline stores. The effects of a single large dose or multiple smaller doses of reserpine were identical, so the results were pooled. In contrast to denervation, reserpine treatment did not significantly alter the response pattern of hypothyroid atria to agonists, and the effects of antagonists also remained unchanged. These results suggest that some factor related to sympathetic nerves other than noradrenaline may be involved in the thyroid-induced shifts in α- and β-receptor responses. Results of ligand binding studies confirmed this conclusion and suggested that the observed effects of sympathetic denervation were mediated by changes in the relative numbers of α- and β-receptor binding sites. Denervation of hypothyroid rats by 6-OHDA increased the density of DHA and decreased the density of WB-4101 binding sites, which resulted in the reversal of the α:β ratio from 1.44 to 0.58. Reserpine treatment had no significant effects on the densities of either α- or β-adrenoceptors (Kunos et al., 1980).

Finally, two questions remain to be discussed: what is the mechanism of thyroid modulation of cardiac adrenoceptors and what is their biological significance. Although reciprocal, matching changes in receptor densities are compatible with an interconversion mechanism, as suggested earlier, they do not directly prove it. Preliminary studies in my laboratory indicate that a small effect of thyroid hormones on receptor densities can be detected as early as after 1 hour of in vitro incubation of hypothyroid heart slices with T_3. These rapid changes, which have been shown to occur in a number of other tissue or cell systems, do not appear to require the synthesis of new receptor protein, and could possibly reflect direct, coupled regulation of α- and β-receptors. Evidence for such direct, inverse coupling has recently been provided for adrenoceptors in rat brain, where a desensitizing concentration of isoproterenol decreased the density of β and increased the density of α_2 receptors which are predominantly postsynaptic in the rat brain, and both changes could be prevented by a β-receptor antagonist (Maggi et al., 1980). Elucidation of the molecular basis for this apparent functional 'interconversion' of adrenoceptors may be expected when the structure and membrane localization of adrenoceptors will be clarified.

Regardless of its molecular mechanism, 'interconversion' of adrenoceptors may have biological significance. β-receptors are usually more sensitive to the same, naturally occurring catecholamine than α-receptors, and a change in their balance may represent a mechanism of regulating the sensitivity of the heart to catecholamines. Such changes may be part of the adaptation of the tissue to altered metabolic conditions. It is also interesting to point out that the minor α-adrenergic component in responses of the normal myocardium may reflect the embryologic development of the heart from vascular tissue. Motor responses of the latter remain to be mediated by α-receptors, whereas the most highly differentiated myocardial cells, the pacemaker cells, do not appear to have any α-receptor component in their rate response to catecholamines. Thyroid hormones are important in cell and tissue differentiation, and their effects in altering the balance between α- and β-receptors may be part of the process of cell differentiation. In line with this speculation, it has been recently reported that α-receptors are present in fetal but not in adult sheep myocardium, and β-receptors showed a reciprocal change with ontogenic development (Cheng et al., 1980).

REFERENCES

Ahlquist, R.P. (1948): A study of adrenotropic receptors. Amer. J. Physiol. <u>183</u>, 586-600.

Cheng, J.B., Cornett, L.E., Goldfin, A. & Roberts, J.M. (1980). α-Adrenergic receptor is present in fetal but not adult sheep myocardium. Fed. Proc. <u>39</u>, 399A.

Guicheney, P., Garay, R.P., Levy-Marchal, C. & Meyer, P. (1978): Biochemical evidence of presynaptic and postsynaptic α-adrenoceptors in rat heart membranes: positive homotropic cooperativity of presynaptic binding. Proc. Natl. Acad. Sci. USA 75, 6285-6289.

Hashimoto, H. & Nakashima, M. (1978): Influence of thyroid hormone on the positive inotropic effects mediated by α-β-adrenoceptors in isolated guinea pig atria and rabbit papillary muscles. Eur. J. Pharmacol. 50, 337-347.

Kunos, G. (1977): Thyroid hormone dependent interconversion of myocardial α- and β-adrenoceptors in the rat. Brit. J. Pharmacol. 59, 177-190.

Kunos, G. (1978): Adrenoceptors. Ann. Rev. Pharmacol. tox. 18, 291-311.

Kunos, G. (1980): Reciprocal changes in α- and β-adrenoceptors - myth or reality? Trends in Pharmacol. Sci. 1, 282-284.

Kunos, G., Hoffman, B., Kwok, Y.N., Kan, W.H. & Mucci, L.: Dihydroergocryptine binding and α-adrenoceptors in smooth muscle. Nature 278, 254-256.

Kunos, G., Mucci, L. & O'Regan, S. (1980): The influence of hormonal and neuronal factors on rat heart adrenoceptors. Br. J. Pharmac. in press.

Kunos, G. & Nickerson, M. (1976): Temperature-induced interconversion of α- and β-adrenoceptors in the frog heart. J. Physiol. (London) 256, 23-40.

Kunos, G. & Preiksaitis, H.G. (1978): Induced changes in adrenoceptor properties. In: Recent advances in the pharmacology of adrenoceptors, ed. by E. Szabadi, C.M. Bradshaw & P. Bevan, Elsevier/North Holland, Amsterdam, p. 209-216.

Kunos, G. & Szentivanyi, M. (1968): Evidence favouring the existence of a single adrenergic receptor. Nature 217, 1077-1078.

Maggi, A., U'Prichard, D.C. & Enna, S.J. (1980): β-Adrenergic regulation of α_2-adrenergic receptors in the central nervous system. Science 207, 645-646.

Nahorski, S.R. & Richardson, A. (1979): Pitfalls in the assessment of the specific binding of (-) ^{3}H-dihydroalprenolol to β-adrenoceptors. Brit. J. Pharmacol. 66, 479-470P.

Nakashima, M., Fsuru, H. & Shigei, T. (1973): Stimulant action of methoxamine in the isolated atria of normal and 6-propyl-2-thiouracil-fed rats. Jap. J. Pharmacol. 23, 307-312.

Nickerson, M. & Kunos, G. (1977): Discussion of evidence regarding induced changes in adrenoceptors. Fed. Proc. 36, 2580-2583.

Schüman, H.J., Endoh, M. & Wagner, J. (1974): Positive isotropic effects of phenylephrine in the isolated rabbit papillary muscle mediated by both α- and β-adrenoceptors. Naunyn Schmiedeberg's Arch. Pharmacol. 284, 133-148.

Winek, R. & Bhalla, R. (1979): ^{3}H-dihydroalprenolol binding sites in rat myocardium: relationship between a single binding site population and the concentration of radioligand. Biophys. Res. Commun. <u>91</u>, 200-206.

Work from the author's laboratory was supported by grants from the Medical Research Council of Canada.

Discussion

<u>Juhász-Nagy</u>: There is a controversy to your data that claims that alpha- and beta-adrenoceptors were not interconvertible and also your experiments with thyroid hormones could be explained by non-interconversion theory. What do you say about it?

<u>Kunos</u>: There are many examples of reciprocal changes in alpha- and beta-receptors and receptor responses. WE also found that chemical sympathectomy with 6-hydroxydopamine shortly after thyreoidectomy, but not depletion of noradrenaline stores with reserpine, prevented the shift from beta- to alpha-receptors. This suggests that in the rat heart a trophic influence of sympathetic innervation not involving normal stores of the neurotransmitter may have a role in maintaining changes in the balance of alpha- and beta-adrenoceptors.

ASPECTS ON THE BETA-1-ADRENOCEPTOR STIMULATORY MECHANISM OF PRENALTEROL

Hillevi Mattsson, Anders Hedberg and Enar Carlsson
AB Hässle, Department of Pharmacology, S-431 83 Mölndal, Sweden

INTRODUCTION

Prenalterol ((-)-H 80/62, H 133/22) has previously been characterized as a selective beta-1-adrenoceptor agonist with about 80 per cent intrinsic activity of that of isoprenaline on heart rate and cardiac contractility in the anaesthetized cat (Carlsson et al. 1977).

For a further characterization of the interaction of prenalterol with beta-adrenoceptors, its effects have been compared with those of isoprenaline and procaterol (OPC 2009) on contractility in cat heart and on subtetanic contractions in soleus muscle in vitro, as well as on beta-adrenoceptor binding and adenylate cyclase activity in those tissues.

Isoprenaline was used as a non-selective full beta-adrenoceptor agonist and procaterol has been reported to be a selective beta-2-adrenoceptor partial agonist (Yabuuchi 1977). Our choice of tissue is based on the finding that the cat ventricles are almost homogeneously supplied with beta-1-adrenoceptors (Hedberg et al. 1980), whereas the subtetanic contractions and twitches in the soleus muscle are controlled by beta-2-adrenoceptors (Waldeck 1976). This tissue has been shown to contain almost no beta-1-adrenoceptors (Minneman et al. 1979 a).

The possible involvement of alpha-adrenoceptor interaction in the inotropic response to prenalterol was studied in rabbit papillary muscle.

METHODS

Cats and rabbits of either sex, pretreated with reserpine (5 mg/kg i.p.) 18 hours prior to pentobarbital anaesthesia (30 mg/kg i.p.) were used.

Cat and rabbit papillary muscles from the right ventricles
were used to study the positive inotropic effect. The muscles
were driven to contract isometrically at 1 Hz (5 msec
duration) by a current 20 % above threshold at 32°C.

Cat soleus muscle strips were used to study the beta-2-
mediated physiological effects. Beta-2-adrenoceptor
stimulation in the soleus muscle results in reduced tension
of the subtetanic contractions due to decreased duration of
the twitches. The method was essentially that described for
whole soleus muscle from guinea pig (Waldeck 1976).

Supramaximal pulses (0.5 msec duration) were delivered in
trains of 1.5 sec duration at about 12 Hz to evoke subtetanic
contractions alternating with single twitches every 10 sec.
The beta-2-stimulatory effect was expressed as the decrease
in force ratio between subtetanic contractions and twitches
(S/T).

Beta-adrenoceptor binding was performed in crude membrane
preparations of ventricular and soleus muscle using [^{125}I]
iodohydroxybenzylpindolol (IHYP) as a labelled ligand
(Minneman et al. 1979a). The Cheng-Prusoff equation (1973)
was used for calculation of K_d values and for construction
of the concentration beta-adrenoceptor occupancy curve for
the compounds.

Adenylate cyclase activity was assayed by measuring the
conversion of alpha [^{32}P]-ATP to alpha [^{32}P]-cyclic AMP in
tissue homogenates of ventricular and soleus muscle
(Minneman et al. 1979b).

RESULTS AND DISCUSSION

The binding experiments with radiolabelled IHYP reveal that
isoprenaline, prenalterol and procaterol displaced all
specifically bound IHYP in both heart (beta-1) and soleus
muscle (beta-2) (Fig. 1) which indicates that all three
agonists bind to both beta-adrenoceptor subtypes. The
negative logarithm of the dissociation constants (pK_d) show
that the beta-adrenoceptor affinities for isoprenaline and
prenalterol are the same in the heart and soleus muscle
(Table 1). The affinity of procaterol was about 2 log units
higher for the beta-2-adrenoceptors in the soleus muscle than
for the cardiac beta-1-adrenoceptors. Hofstee analysis
(Minneman et al. 1979a) of the inhibition of specific IHYP
binding by procaterol implies that a minor fraction of the
beta-adrenoceptors in the heart show the same affinity for
the drug as the beta-2-receptors in the soleus muscle.

Isoprenaline increased the adenylate cyclase activity about
5-fold in the heart and 6-fold in the soleus muscle
preparation. Prenalterol and procaterol induced only a
marginal, however, not statistically significant, elevation
of the adenylate cyclase activity in the heart. In the

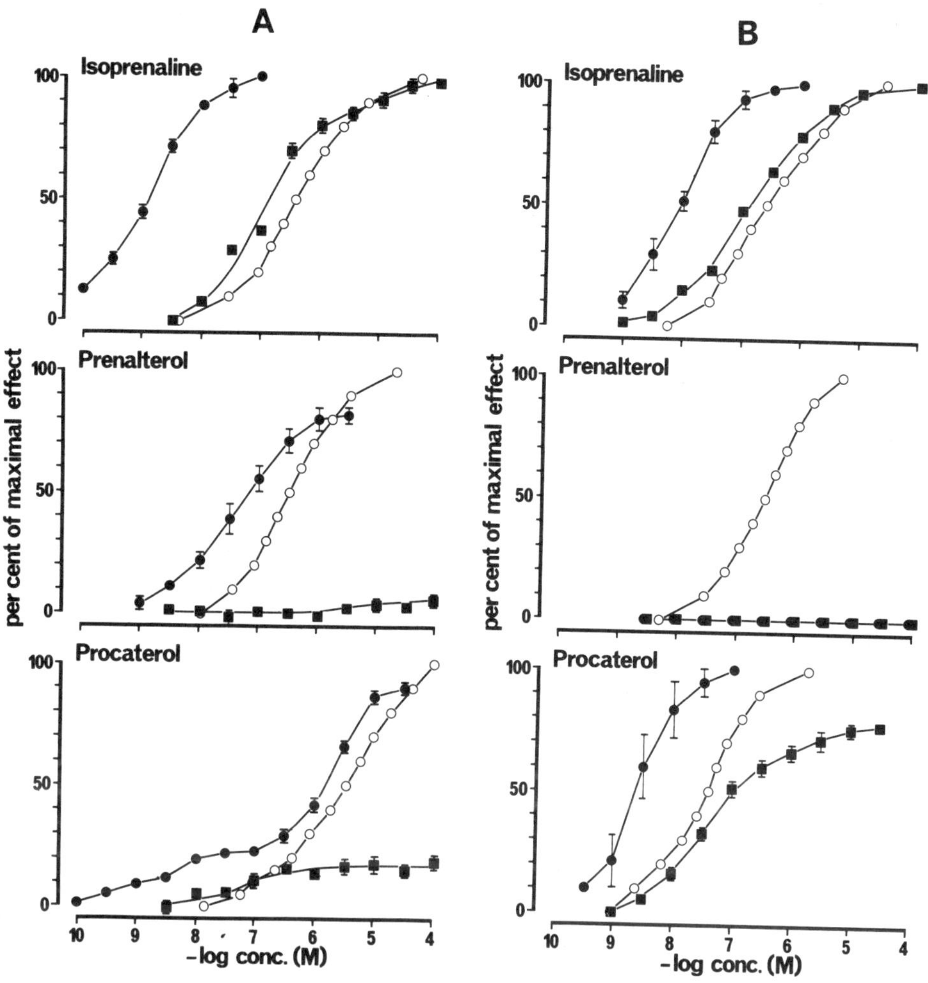

Fig. 1. Concentration effect curves for isoprenaline, prenalterol and procaterol in cat ventricular myocardium (A) and soleus muscle (B). Effects on muscle contractions (●), adenylate cyclase activity (■) and beta-adrenoceptor occupancy (○) are expressed in per cent of maximal effect of isoprenaline and plotted versus the negative logarithm of the concentrations. Bars indicate SEM (n ≥ 6).

soleus muscle preparation prenalterol was totally devoid of stimulatory effect, whereas procaterol increased the adenylate cyclase activity to 77 per cent of that of isoprenaline (Fig. 1).

In cat papillary muscle isoprenaline and prenalterol displayed monophasic concentration effect curve for the

<u>Table 1.</u> Affinity values (-log mean ± SEM) for beta-
adrenoceptors derived from IHYP-binding in cat heart and
soleus muscle (n = 6).

	Cat ventricle pK_d	Cat soleus muscle pK_d
Isoprenaline	6.48 ± 0.11	6.31 ± 0.10
Prenalterol	6.38 ± 0.07	6.37 ± 0.15
Procaterol		
beta-1	5.18 ± 0.07	−
beta-2	7.03 ± 0.19	7.17 ± 0.04

positive inotropic response (Fig. 1). The maximal
contractility effect of prenalterol was 82 ± 3 per cent of
that of isoprenaline (n = 7). Procaterol on the other hand
induced a biphasic effect curve for the contractility response
(Fig. 1). The high and low affinity curve components were
due to activation of beta-2- and beta-1-adrenoceptors,
respectively, since they were selectively blocked by the beta-
2-antagonist IPS 339 (0.03 µM) and the beta-1-antagonist
pamatolol (0.6 µM) (Imbs et al. 1977, Carlsson et al. 1976).
The beta-2-adrenoceptor mediated effect amounted to 23 ± 3
per cent and the total tension induced by procaterol was
92 ± 2 per cent of that of isoprenaline (n = 15).

The relationship between the effects of isoprenaline
stimulation on the contractile force and on adenylate cyclase
activity or beta-adrenoceptor occupancy in the heart revealed
a hundred-fold separation. It is evident that only about
10-20 per cent of the beta-adrenoceptors have to be occupied
by isoprenaline to achieve the maximal contractile response.
These data support the spare receptor theory (Kaumann 1978)
and predict a beta-adrenoceptor reserve amounting to 80-90 per
cent for a full agonist in the cat myocardium. For the
partial agonist prenalterol and for procaterol in its low
affinity range the concentration effect curves for
contractility and receptor occupancy are far more fused. The
maximal positive inotropic effects of prenalterol and
procaterol are achieved at about 80 and 90 per cent receptor
occupancy, respectively (Fig. 1).

The isoprenaline data also reveal that the maximal
contractility effect is obtained at only about 30 per cent of
the total adenylate cyclase activation. Possibly the marginal
increases in adenylate cyclase activity induced by prenalterol
and procaterol in the heart are sufficient to achieve the
maximal contractility effects of those compounds. The
involvement of the adenylate cyclase-cyclic AMP system in the
mediation of the physiological responses by beta-1-
adrenoceptors may, however, have to be questioned.

In the soleus muscle strips isoprenaline and procaterol
decreased the force ratio between the subtetanic contractions
and twitches to the same extent, 32 ± 3 (n = 8) and 30 ± 6
(n = 5) per cent, respectively. The concentration effect
curves for contraction response and receptor occupancy are
separated for both agonists in the skeletal muscle indicating
a beta-2-adrenoceptor reserve of 30 - 50 per cent. In this
tissue the maximal effect on the subtetanic contractions was
obtained at about 65 - 75 per cent adenylate cyclase
activation. Prenalterol was devoid of effect on adenylate
cyclase activity as well as on subtetanic contractions in the
soleus muscle strips. Prenalterol thus binds to the
adrenoceptors in the skeletal muscle but lacks intrinsic beta-
2 agonistic activity.

In the rabbit papillary muscle prenalterol induced a positive
inotropic response which in the presence of the beta-1
antagonist metoprolol (0.3 µM) was shifted to the right,
whereas the alpha-blocker phentolamine (1.0 µM) did not
antagonize the response (Fig. 2) This indicates that the
contractility effect by prenalterol in the heart is mediated
via beta-1-adrenoceptors and that alpha-adrenoceptors are not
involved. In the presence of phentolamine there was, however,
a tendency towards an increased apparent affinity for
prenalterol. A similar tendency has also been observed for
other beta-adrenoceptor agonists at alpha-blockade and
requires further investigation.

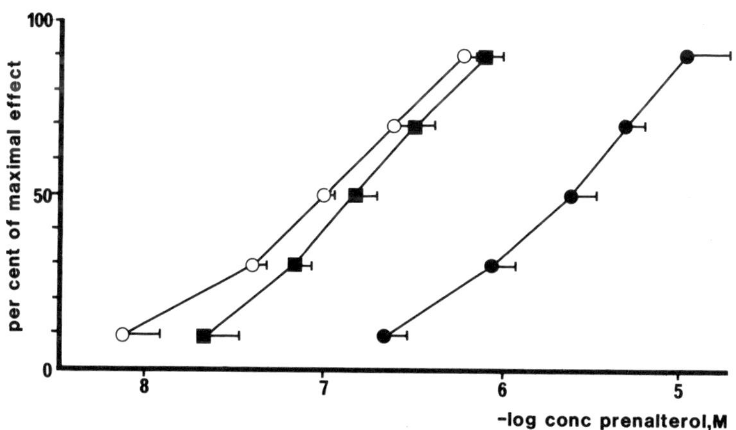

Fig. 2. Concentration effect curves for the positive
inotropic effect in rabbit papillary muscle of prenalterol
in the absence (■) and in the presence of metoprolol 0.3 µM
(●) or phentolamine 1.0 µM (○) n = 4.

CONCLUSIONS

Prenalterol binds to both beta-1- and beta-2-adrenoceptors
with equal affinity. The cardio-selective effect of
prenalterol is due to the fact that prenalterol has intrinsic
stimulatory activity only on beta-1-adrenoceptors. Alpha-
adrenoceptors do not seem to be involved in the positive
inotropic response induced by prenalterol.

The cardiac inotropic effect of prenalterol is achieved at
low, if any, increase of adenylate cyclase activity. This
finding may indicate that there is a large receptor and
adenylate cyclase activity reserve for full agonists in the
cardiac muscle. Consequently, a marginal increase in the
adenylate cyclase activity might be sufficient to achieve the
maximal contractility effect of prenalterol. The lack of
adenylate cyclase activation might also be due to the fact
that the inotropic response of a beta-1-adrenoceptor partial
agonist such as prenalterol is not mediated via cyclic AMP.

REFERENCES

Carlsson, E., Ek, L., Lundgren, B. and Åblad, B. (1976)
Pharmacological investigations with H 104/08. Investigators
Brochure. Haessle Pharmaceuticals, Göteborg, Sweden.

Carlsson, E., Dahlöf, C.-G., Hedberg, A., Persson, H. and
Tångstrand, B. (1977)
Differentiation of cardiac chronotropic and inotropic effects
of β-adrenoceptor agonists. Naunyn-Schmiedeberg´s Arch.
Pharmacol. $\underline{300}$:101-105.

Cheng, Y.-C. and Prusoff, W.H. (1973)
Relationship between the inhibition constant (K_i) and the
concentration of inhibitor which causes a 50 percent inhibition
(IC_{50}) of an enzyme reaction. Biochem. Pharmacol. $\underline{22}$:3099-3108.

Hedberg, A., Minneman, K.P. and Molinoff, P.B. (1980)
Differential distribution of beta-1 and beta-2 adrenergic
receptors in cat and guinea pig heart. J. Pharmacol. Exp.
Ther. $\underline{212}$:503-508.

Imbs, J.L., Miesch, F., Schwartz, J., Velly, J., Leclerc, G.,
Mann, A. and Wermuth, C.G. (1977)
A potent new β_2-adrenoceptor blocking agent. Br. J. Pharmacol.
$\underline{60}$:357-362.

Kaumann, A.J. (1978)
On spare β-adrenoceptors for inotropic effects of catechola-
mines in kitten ventricle. Naunyn-Schmiedeberg´s Arch.
Pharmacol. $\underline{305}$:97-102.

Minneman, K.P., Hedberg, A. and Molinoff, P.B. (1979 a)
Comparison of beta adrenergic receptor subtypes in mammalian
tissues. J. Pharmacol. Exp. Ther. $\underline{211}$:502-508.

Minneman, K.P., Hegstrand, L.R. and Molinoff, P.B. (1979 b)
The pharmacological specificity of β_1 and β_2-adrenergic
receptors in the rat heart and lung in vitro. Mol. Pharmacol.
16:21-33.

Waldeck, B. (1976)
An in vitro method for the study of β-receptor mediated
effects on slow contracting skeletal muscle. J. Pharm.
Pharmacol. 28:434-436.

Yabuuchi, Y. (1977)
The β-adrenoceptor stimulant properties of OPC-2009 on guinea-
pig isolated tacheal, right atrial and left atrial preparations. Br. J. Pharmacol. 61:513-521.

DISCUSSION OF PAPER

Dr G. Kunos: Your results are very interesting. I think they
represent the first demonstration that in the heart adenylate
cyclase may be selectively associated with beta-2-receptors.
Is it possible that the phenomenon of receptor reserve for
beta-receptors is simply a reflection of the proportion of
beta-1-receptors in a system?

Dr H. Mattsson: It also appears that the beta-1 and beta-2
adrenoceptor mediated adenylate cyclase activation in the
heart is subject to compartmentation since the level of
adenylate cyclase activation observed in the beta-2 affinity
range of procaterol exceeds that of prenalterol (beta-1)
although the inotropic effect induced by procaterol in that
range is less than 1/3 of the total contractility response
to prenalterol.

Since our data are derived only from heart and soleus muscle,
it is not valid to make extrapolations about receptor reserve
to other tissues. The cardiac response pattern of procaterol
in the beta-2 affinity range may, however, imply that a spare
beta-2-adrenoceptor pool exists in the heart, similar to that
described for the soleus muscle. Possibly the beta-adrenoceptor subtypes display characteristics which are similar in
various organs so that the spare beta-1 adrenoceptor pool is
80-90 % and the spare beta-2-pool is 30-50 % of total,
regardless of the tissue. This hypothesis implies that the
relation beta-1/beta-2 in an organ determines the net amount
of spare receptors observed.

Dr G. Kunos: What is the reason for the fact that prenalterol
is highly selective for beta-1-receptors when physiological
responses are measured, but lacks selectivity in binding
assays, as the K_d´s for binding to beta-1 and beta-2 were
identical.

Dr H. Mattsson: Our data indicate that prenalterol has
stimulatory activity only on beta-1-adrenoceptors, but lacks
this property on beta-2-adrenoceptors. Whether this stimulatory mechanism involves the coupling of receptor to adenylate

cyclase is uncertain, but the deficiency of physiological activity appears to be associated with a lack of adequate cyclase activation. Prenalterol has been shown to be a competitive antagonist of isoprenaline in the soleus muscle, thus demonstrating its ability to bind to beta-2-adrenoceptors in addition to beta-1.

<u>Dr R.A. Riemersma</u>: Is prenalterol taken up into the synaptic vesicles of the heart?

<u>Dr H. Mattsson</u>: The affinity of prenalterol for cardiac beta-adrenoceptors was found in the contractility experiments to be unaltered in the presence of 5 µM cocaine. Therefore, the compound does not appear to be taken up into presynaptic structures.

<u>Dr R.A. Riemersma</u>: Is it possible that the apparent dissociation between the effect of isoprenaline and prenalterol on the relation between cAMP and inotropism is accounted for by a difference in their effects on phosphodiesterase?

<u>Dr H. Mattsson</u>: In our adenylate cyclase activity assays <u>in vitro</u> the phosphodiesterase inhibitor IBMX was always present and any differences in the effect of prenalterol and isoprenaline on phosphodiesterase was eliminated. Thus, when the <u>in vitro</u> adenylate cyclase activity data are correlated to inotropic responses, phosphodiesterase activation is unlikely to affect the interrelation between the two variables.

ON THE MECHANISM
OF ADENOSINE-INDUCED INHIBITION
OF ADRENERGIC NEUROTRANSMISSION
IN THE VENTRICULAR MYOCARDIUM OF
GUINEA PIGS

A. J. Szentmiklósi, Ágnes Cseppentő and J. Szegi
Department of Pharmacology, University Medical School, Debrecen, H-4012 Debrecen, Hungary

There is increasing evidence in the literature indicating
that adenosine modulates adrenergic neurotransmission in a
number of tissues. Adenosine has been shown to inhibit the
nerve stimulated release of noradrenaline in vas deferens
/Hedquist and Fredholm 1976; Clanachan et al. 1977; Muller
and Paton 1979/, in perfused adipose tissue and kidney /Hed-
quist and Fredholm 1976/, as well as in blood vessels
/Verhaeghe et al. 1977; Enero and Saidman 1977/. On the other
hand, it appears to facilitate the neurally mediated noradrenaline release of the spleen /Mueller et al. 1979/.

Only in the past few years has it become apparent that
such a mechanism may also exist also for the heart. Hedquist
and Fredholm were the first -in 1979- to describe the inhibitory effect of adenosine on adrenergic neuroeffector transmission of the isolated perfused rabbit heart. It was also
shown in the same year /Lokhandwala 1979a; Juhász-Nagy et al.
1979/ that adenosine was capable of inhibiting the cardiac
sympathetic neurotransmission of dog hearts also under in
vivo conditions. Quite recently Khan and Malik /1980/ have
described that adenosine inhibited the K^+-evoked release of
/^3H/-noradrenaline from rat heart slices.

In a previous study /Szentmiklósi et al. 1979/ we showed
that adenosine was also capable of significantly reducing the
mechanical responses elicited by electrical field stimulation
on isolated, electrically driven right papillary muscles of
guinea pigs -on preparations, where the accidental haemo-

dynamic and chronotropic influence of interfering character
elicited by adenosine could probably be avoided. The purpose
of our present investigation was to study in detail the character of this modulatory action.

METHODS AND MATERIALS

Guinea pigs of either sex were killed by a blow on the
head. The papillary muscles with a diameter of less than 1 mm
were dissected from the right ventricles and suspended in a
75-ml tissue bath containing Krebs solution of the following
composition /mmol/l/: NaCl, 118; KCl, 4.7; $CaCl_2$, 2.5;
NaH_2PO_4, 1.0; $MgCl_2$, 1.2; $NaHCO_3$, 24.9 and glucose 11.5 equilibrated with 95% O_2 and 5% CO_2. The temperature of the solution was maintained at 37^OC /pH 7.4/. Atropine sulphate at a
concentration of 0.1 μmol/l was added to the nutrient solution
to prevent any effect of acetylcholine released by electrical
field stimulation /Blinks 1966/. Resting force was adjusted
to obtain maximal contractions. The muscles were driven electrically via platinum electrodes at a rate of 2 Hz /unless
otherwise stated/ by square wave electrical impulses of 1 ms
duration with the technique described by Blinks /1966/ slightly modified by Vizi et al. /1973/. Punctate platinum electrodes
were used to deliver threshold stimuli throughout the experiments. Another platinum electrode was placed near the muscle
for field stimulation. The intensity of the field stimuli was
supramaximal and their duration and frequency were the same
as those of the threshold stimuli. The number of field pulses
was varied from 10 to 320 shocks. The stimulation periods were
separated by intervals of 4 min. The increase of contractile
tension in response to field stimulation as used in the present
experiments could be abolished by pindolol /0.1 μmol/l/, a
beta-adrenergic receptor blocking agent or could be prevented
by in vivo reserpine pretreatment /5 mg/kg i.p. one day before
the experiment/.

The muscles were equilibrated for 1 to 2 hours until
contractile force and response to field stimulation /80 shocks/

reached a maximum and steady level. Mechanical responses were
displayed on an oscilloscope /EMG 1555 TR-4653/ and recorded
on film or polygraph.

The data were evaluated by Student's test for paired data
by means of a table calculator /PTK-1072/.

The substances used were: adenosine, inosine /Boehringer,
Mannheim/, hypoxanthine /Reanal, Budapest/, aminophylline,
noradrenaline bitartrate, reserpine /Richter, Budapest/ atro-
pine sulphate /EGYT, Budapest/, phentolamine methansulphonate
/CIBA-GEIGY, Basle/, phenoxybenzamine /TCI, Tokyo/, indometha-
cin /Sigma, St. Louis/, dipyridamole /VEB Arzneimittelwerke,
Dresden/. The adenosine deaminase /adenosine aminohydrolase,
E.C. 3.5.4.4/ from calf intestinal mucosa was purchased from
Boehringer /Mannheim/ as a suspension in glycerol /specific
activity: 200 U/mg/. The metiamide was a generous gift from
Smith Kline and French Labs. Ltd. /Welwyn Garden City/.

RESULTS

1. <u>Effect of adenosine on the mechanical responses of papillary muscles to electrical field stimulation</u>

The mechanical responses of papillary muscles to field
stimulation depended on the number of pulses when a frequency
of 2 Hz was used and the increase of contractions was maximal
or near maximal at 160 shocks /Fig. 1/. These mechanical responses to field stimulation were significantly reduced in the
presence of adenosine /10 μmol/-1 mmol/l; n = 17/. Adenosine
at relatively low concentrations /1-10 μmol/l/ had no effect
on the contractile tension by itself, whereas, at higher concentrations it exerted a slight positive inotropic action
/about 5-12% above controls/. Fig. 2 shows the percent of
inhibitions elicited by adenosine at 80 shocks /a number of
field pulses inducing a nearly half-maximal response to field
stimulation/. It should be noted that the inhibitory action
of adenosine was virtually independent on the number of field
pulses.

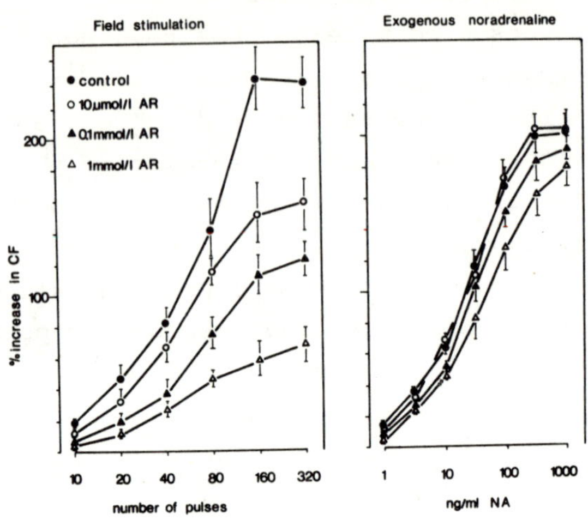

Fig. 1   Effects of adenosine of responses of guinea pig ventricular myocardium to electrical field stimulation /n=17/
and to exogenous noradrenaline /n=14/. All results are
expressed as % increase in contractile force $^{\pm}$ S.E.M.
AR: adenosine; NA: noradrenaline; CF: contractile force

2. Influence of adenosine on contractile response to exogenous noradrenaline

In the analysis of the possible site of action of a substance modulating adrenergic neurotransmission, the first ap-
roach widely used is to compare its effects on responses to
nerve stimulation and exogenous noradrenaline. Therefore, experiments were performed to reveal whether adenosine was able
to influence the action of exogenously applied noradrenaline
on the mechanical activity of guinea pig papillary muscles.
Fig. 1 shows that adenosine at concentrations of 10 μmol/l-
-1 mmol/l caused only a slight reduction in the increase of

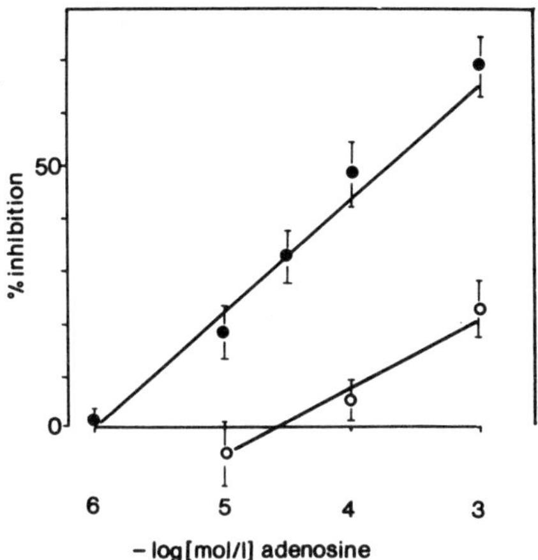

Fig. 2 Influence of adenosine on responses of guinea pig
           papillary muscles to field stimulation /80 shocks/
           and to exogenous norepinephrine /30 ng/ml/. Results
           are expressed as mean inhibition $\pm$ S.E.M.

mechanical activity of papillary muscles in response to exogenous noradrenaline /1 ng/ml-1µg/ml/. Fig. 2 demonstrates that
adenosine is about 100 times stronger /measured at 20% inhibi-
tion/ in inhibiting the response to electrical field stimulation than exogenously applied noradrenaline, which indicates
a predominantly presynaptic site of action for this purine nucleoside.

3. Influence of the blockade of muscarinic receptors

The inhibitory effect of adenosine at a concentration of
100 µmol/l /a concentration of this nucleoside inducing a nearly
half-maximal inhibition in response to electrical field stimulation at 80 shocks/ on the mechanical responses to field stimuli was unchanged both in the absence or in the presence of atropine sulphate /0.1 µmol/l/; the percent inhibitions by adenosine /100 µmol/l/ were 46.2 $\pm$ 3.7 and 48.9 $\pm$ 4.6 /n=4/, respec-

Table I

<u>Involvement of presynaptic receptors in the adenosine-induced
inhibition of responses of ventricular myocardium to electrical field stimulation</u>

Treatment	% inhibition of mechanical responses	
	in the absence	in the presence of the blocking agent
Phenoxybenzamine 0.1 μmol/l; n=5	51.7 $\pm$ 6.7	47.9 $\pm$ 5.5 n. s.
Phentolamine 1 μmol/l; n=6	46.7 $\pm$ 5.8	48.6 $\pm$ 5.9 n. s.
Metiamide 1 μmol/l; n=4	43.2 $\pm$ 3.7	42.5 $\pm$ 2.8 n. s.
Indomethacin 2.8 μmol/l; n=6	53.2 $\pm$ 1.7	42.7 $\pm$ 2.6 $p < 0.01$

p: represents the significance of the difference from
   the inhibition in untreated tissues.
n. s.:/p>0.1/

tively /p>0.1/. However, in order to prevent any possible interfering effect of acetylcholine released during electrical
field stimulation, the nutrient solution was completed with
atropine sulphate /0.1 μmol/l/ throughout the experimental
procedures.

4. <u>Effects of the blockade of alfa-adrenergic and H_2 histamine</u>
   <u>receptors</u>

In order to exclude the possible involvement of presynaptic alfa-adrenergic and H_2 histamine receptors in the inhibitory potency of adenosine in the adrenergic neurotransmission
of the heart, experiments were made also in the presence of
alfa-adrenergic blocking drugs -phenoxybenzamine /0.1 µmol/l/
and phentolamine /1 µmol/l/- as well as under the blockade of
H_2 histamine receptors by metiamide / 1 µmol/l/.

As Table I indicates, neither the blockade of alfa-adrenergic receptors nor that of H_2 histamine receptors was able to
influence significantly the percent inhibitory action of adenosine on the increase in contractile force elicited by field
stimulation.

5. <u>Involvement of prostaglandins in the inhibitory effect of</u>
   <u>adenosine</u>

Adenosine has been proved to stimulate the liberation of
prostaglandins /Needleman et al. 1974; Zehl et al. 1976/. To analyse the possible implication of prostaglandins -which may inhibit adrenergic neurotransmission at a presynaptic site of action /Illés et al. 1973; Hedquist 1974; Hadházy et al. 1976;
Hadházy and Nádor 1976/- in the inhibitory action of adenosine
on the neurochemical transmission, in vitro pretreatments were
undertaken with indomethacin /inhibitor of prostaglandin syn-
thesis/ at a relatively low concentration /2.8 µmol/l/. Sur-
prisingly, the presence of indomethacin significantly attenuated
/by 19.6%/ the adenosine-induced reduction in the contractile
responses of papillary muscles to field stimulation /Table I/.

6. <u>Effect of aminophylline</u>

Aminophylline and theophylline as competitive antagonists
of adenosine in a number of tissues are extensively used substances in revealing the possible involvement of P_1 purinergic
receptors in different physiological processes /Burnstock 1972,
1976, 1978/. In the experiments presented here aminophylline
/200 µmol/l/ was capable of significantly reducing, or even
virtually abolishing the inhibitory action of adenosine on the

mechanical effects of electrical field stimuli in ventricular myocardium of guinea pigs /Table II/.

Table II

<u>Role of presynaptic P_1 purinoceptors in the adenosine-induced inhibitory action on responses of guinea pig papillary muscles to field stimulation</u>

	% inhibition of mechanical responses	
Treatment	in the absence	in the presence of the drug
Aminophylline 200 µmol/l; n=7	46.7 ± 3.9	1.2 ± 2.3 $p < 0.001$
Adenosine deaminase 5 µg/ml; n=8	50.2 ± 3.9	-4.6 ± 5.9 $p < 0.001$
Dipyridamole 0.3 µmol/l; n=5	49.4 ± 4.1	68.7 ± 3.5 $p < 0.01$

p: represents the significance of the difference from the inhibition in untreated tissues.

7. Effect of adenosine deaminase

When the mechanical responses to field stimulation were depressed by adenosine, adenosine deaminase /5µg/ml/ added to the nutrient solution restored the responses to the control level /Table II/. Adenosine deaminase is thought to be an enzyme converting adenosine to inosine. In this way, addition of adenosine deaminase to the organ bath could abolish the direct action of adenosine.

8. <u>Influence of degradation products of adenosine on responses</u>
<u>to the field stimulation of ventricular myocardium</u>

The possible involvement of two degradative products of
adenosine /inosine and hypoxanthine/ was studied in the adenosine-induced depression of adrenergic neuroeffector transmission. Neither inosine nor hypoxanthine at a concentrations of
100 μmol/l, was able to alter significantly the increase in
mechanical responses to the field stimulation of papillary
muscles. The percent changes in responses to field stimulation in the presence of inosine or hypoxanthine at the above
concentration were 3.3 $\pm$ 7.3 and 6.7 $\pm$ 7.1, respectively
/p>0.1/.

9. <u>Effect of dipyridamole</u>

Dipyridamole has been reported to inhibit the cellular uptake of adenosine in various tissues /Kübler et al. 1970; Kolassa et al. 1970; Olsson et al. 1972, 1973; Schrader et al.
1972/, so this substance is able to potentiate the physiological actions of adenosine /see Burnstock 1972, 1976, 1980/.
The mechanism underlying this potentiation phenomenon might be
attributed to an extracellular accumulation of this nucleoside
due to the inhibition of its intracellular uptake, thus a larger
quantity of adenosine would be available to act on the specific
P_1 purinoceptors on the outer surface of the cell membrane. As
a result of present experiments by incubating the tissues with
dipyridamole at a concentration of 0.3 μmol/l, it was obtained
evidence that this blocking drug of the adenosine uptake mechanism significantly enhanced the suppressing action of adenosine on responses due to field stimulation of guinea pig papillary muscles /Table II/.

10. <u>Relation between external calcium concentration and the in-</u>
<u>hibitory action of adenosine</u>

Adenosine has been shown to reduce the influx of calcium
from the extracellular space, at least in heart muscle /Schra-
der et al. 1975; Belardinelli et al. 1979/ and vascular smooth
muscle /Herlihy et al. 1976/. On the other hand, the inhibitory

action of some presynaptically acting modulators can be influenced by the variation of external calcium concentration /West-
fall and Leighton 1976; Leighton and Westfall 1976/.

The ability of external calcium concentration to modify the
effects of adenosine on responses due to field stimulation was
also examined in present experiments. Fig. 3 shows that the lowering of extracellular Ca^{2+} from 2.5 /normally present in the
nutrient solution/ to 1.25 mmol/l resulted in an enhancement of
the inhibitory potency of adenosine. On the contrary, raising
the external Ca^{2+} concentration to 10 mmol/l near by completely
prevented the inhibition elicited by adenosine /100 µmol/l/.

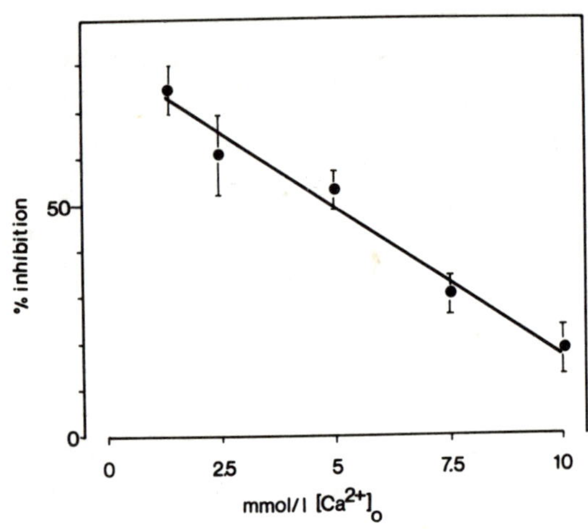

Fig. 3 Calcium-dependent inhibitory action of adenosine
/100 µmol/l/ on responses of guinea pig ventricular
myocardium to electrical field stimulation /80 shocks/
Results are expressed as mean inhibition $\pm$ S.E.M.
n = 6

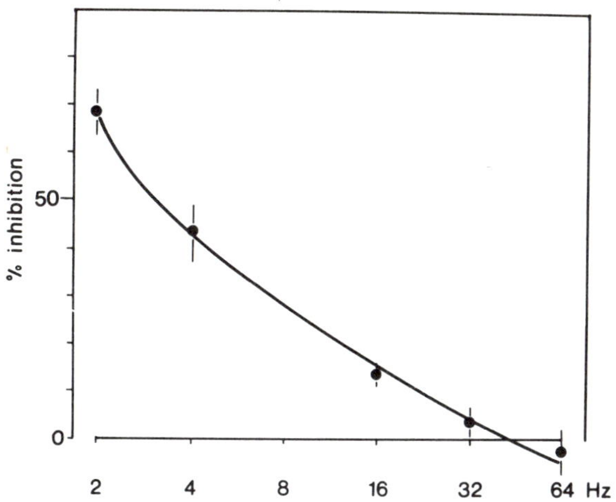

Fig. 4   Frequency-dependent inhibitory action of adenosine in
         responses of guinea pig papillary muscles to electrical
         field stimulation. Results are expressed as mean inhibi-
         tion $\pm$ S.E.M; n = 5

11. <u>Frequency dependence in the action of adenosine</u>

It has been established that reduction in the stimulation
evoked release of noradrenaline by several presynaptically acting substances /alfa-adrenergic agonists, prostaglandins/ is
the more pronounced the lower the frequency of nerve stimulation. At high frequencies, however, these substances fail to
reduce the output of noradrenaline induced by nerve stimulation
/Starke et al. 1975; Langer et al. 1975; Westfall and Leighton
1976; Westfall 1977/.

To analyse whether or not there exists such a frequency-
dependent phenomenon for adenosine, experiments were also performed at a wide range of frequency of field stimulation
/2-4-16-32-64 Hz/. It should be noted that the number of field
pulses of each train was kept constant /80 shocks/. Field
impulses higher than 8 Hz were applied well within the effec-

tive refractory periods of muscles /up to every 65 ms from the
starting of electrical stimulation/ so as to prevent any direct
action on myocardial contractility. The statistical evaluation
of the dependence of the inhibitory action of adenosine on the
frequency of field impulses is depicted in Fig. 4.

Similarly to the above results obtained with calcium, the
adenosine-induced inhibition of mechanical responses to field
stimulation is inversely related to the frequency of field pulses.

DISCUSSION

The experiments presented here have demonstrated that adenosine is an about 100 times more potent inhibitor of responses
to electrical field stimulation than of responses to exogenous
noradrenaline in isolated, electrically driven right papillary
muscles of guinea pigs. These findings are virtually identical
to those obtained for rat vas deferens /Clanachan et al. 1977;
Muller and Paton 1979/ and canine blood vessels /Verhaeghe et
al. 1977/ as well as for dog hearts /Lokhandwala 1979a/.

The fact that adenosine produced only a little effect on
the responses to exogenous noradrenaline suggests that this purine nucleoside can inhibit the adrenergic neurotransmission
of the myocardium via a predominantly prejunctional site of
action. These results are in good agreement with direct studies
of adenosine action on noradrenaline overflow in response to
nerve stimulation. Adenosine has been shown to inhibit to stim-
ulus-induced noradrenaline-release in guinea pig /Hedquist and
Fredholm 1976/ and rat vas deferens /Clanachan et al. 1977/, in
rat portal vein /Enero and Saidman 1977/ and in canine blood
vessels /Verhaeghe et al. 1977/ as well as in rabbit hearts
/Hedquist and Fredholm 1979/.

As the presence of a number a presynaptic receptor mechanisms on postganglionic nerve endings has been described by
various investigators /see Westfall 1977; Starke et al. 1977;
Hedquist and Fredholm 1976; Paton 1979a, 1979b, Lokhandwala
1979b; Burnstock 1980/ the possible involvement of presynaptic

muscarinic, alfa-adrenergic and H_2 histamine receptors in this
action was examined using specific blocking substances of these
receptors. Neither atropine, phenoxybenzamine, phentolamine
nor metiamide were capable of significantly influencing the
inhibitory potency of adenosine on mechanical responses to e-
lectrical field stimulation.

Adenosine is thought to stimulate the liberation of endogenous prostaglandins /Needleman et al. 1974; Zehl et al 1976/.
As the latter could produce presynaptic inhibition, to exclude
the involvement of endogenous prostaglandins in the adenosine
action, in vitro pretreatment of tissues with low concentration
of indomethacin /2.8 µmol/l/ was performed. Preincubation
with indomethacin slightly, but significantly reduced the inhibitory potency of adenosine, suggesting that the liberation
of prostaglandins might be responsible -at least in part- for
the inhibition elicited by adenosine. However, some care should
be taken when considering these data, because indomethacin at
higher concentrations may have exerted effects other than the
inhibition of prostaglandin synthetase /e.g. blockade of nor-
adrenaline-reuptake, depressant action on Ca^{2+} uptake; Clarenbach et al. 1976; Northover 1971/. Moreover, our findings are
inconsistent with the literary data according to which the inhibition of prostaglandin synthetase did not change the inhibitory action of adenosine, at least in vas deferens /Hedquist
and Fredholm 1976; Clanachan et al. 1977; Muller and Paton
1979/ or rat heart slices /Khan and Malik 1980/. Therefore,
further, more detailed studies are required to analyse the
role of prostaglandins in this effect.

Based on the present study suggesting an antagonistic effect of aminophylline /a competitive inhibitor of adenosine
in various tissues/ and a potentiative action of dipyridamole
/a potent inhibitor of the cellular adenosine uptake mechanism/,
as well as an abolishing action of adenosine deaminase /an enzyme converting adenosine to inosine/ on the inhibitory effect
of adenosine in adrenergic neurotransmission, it can be concluded that the influence of this nucleoside on responses to
electrical field stimulation can be due to the direct activ-

ation of prejunctional P_1 purinoceptors. These results are similar to those previously observed in vas deferens /Clanachan et al. 1977; Muller and Paton 1979/, blood vessels /Verhaeghe et al. 1977/ and hearts /Lokhandwala 1979a; Khan and Malik 1979/.

To approach the mechanism of adenosine action on responses to field stimulation, experiments were conducted at different external calcium concentrations in the nutrient solution. It is generally accepted that calcium plays a critical role in the secretory processes of presynaptic nerve terminale /see Blaustein 1979/. On the other hand, a number of presynaptically acting substances /agonists of muscarinic and alfa-adrenergic receptors, prostaglandins/ have been suggested to limit the availability of Ca^{2+} available for secretion /see Westfall 1977/. Our present results in cardiac tissue are consistent with this "calcium hypothesis", for the inhibitory potency of adenosine varied inversely with the concentration of calcium in the nutrient solution.

It has been established that the inhibitory action of prostaglandins and alfa-adrenergic agonists is a function of stimulation parameters. The inhibitory potency of prostaglandins has been shown to be inversely related to the number of pulses in each stimulus train /Illés et al. 1973; Knoll et al. 1975; Stjärne 1979/. On the contrary, the present findings demonstrated that no such phenomenon exists for the inhibitory effect of adenosine in ventricular myocardium. In addition, it is known that the inhibitory potency of prostaglandins, muscarinic and alfa-adrenergic agonist depend on the frequency of field stimulation. Inhibition is maximal at low frequencies of stimulation, whereas it is lost at high stimulation frequencies /Illés et al. 1973; Frame and Hedquist 1975; Leighton and Westfall 1976; Hadházy et al. 1976; Westfall 1977; Stjärne 1979/. This above-mentioned frequency dependence was also true of adenosine-induced inhibition studied in the present experiments. The increasing frequencies of stimulation have been shown to increase the influx of calcium into smooth muscle and into giant squid axon /Baker 1972/. It is of interest, that adenosine is capable of inhibiting calcium influx in different tissues such as in atrial myocardium /Schrader et al. 1975; Belardinelli et al. 1979/ and in vascular smooth muscle /Herlihy et al. 1976/. A similar type of action may also exist for the neural tissue, so the data presented here can also be explained by assuming that the activation of prejunctional P_1 purinoceptors limits the availability of Ca^{2+} available for secretion similarly to that of other prejunctional receptors of inhibitory character.

After all, our data concerning the analysis of adenosine action should, of course, be viewed with some caution because they were obtained without direct measurements of noradrenaline outflow. On the other hand, it must be emphasized that this study was performed at such a concentration of adenosine, at which the inhibitory activity of this nucleoside at postsynaptic site on exogenous noradrenaline was virtually negligible, therefore the present way of our experiments, as a first approach, might be regarded as a viable method for the analysis of pre-synaptic action, as well.

With regard to adenosine the critical question, whether or not this nucleoside released by endogenous source may influence the adrenergic neurotransmission of the heart, remains to be elucidated. Another problem of great importance is whether or not high enough concentration of adenosine are reached at the synaptic cleft of adrenergic nerve terminals in the heart. The fact is that the adenosine concentration of the myocardium can be elevated associated with an inadequate myocardial oxygen supply /Berne 1963; Rubio and Berne 1969; Olsson 1970; Berne and Rubio 1974/ and a relatively high level of its concentration can be reached in the myocardium under certain conditions /Degenring et al. 1975; Thomas et al. 1975/. An evidence of great importance has been reported very recently by Burns tock /1980/, who presented morphological evidence for the existence of purinergic nerves in the atrial muscle of guinea pigs. In such conditions the regulatory function of adenosine in the adrenergic neurotransmission of the heart might be supposed, but a great deal of further studies is required to clarify its importance in the regulation of myocardial functions under physiological and pathological conditions.

This work was supported by the Scientific Research Council, Ministry of Public Health, Hungary, Grant No. 2-06-0101-02-2/Sz

REFERENCES

BAKER, P. F. /1972/ Transport and metabolism of calcium ions in nerve. Progr. Biophys.Mol. Biol. $\underline{24}$, 177-223

BELARDINELLI, L., RUBIO, R. and BERNE, R.M. /1979/ Blockade of Ca^{2+} dependent rat atrial slow action potentials by adenosine and lanthanum. Pflügers Arch. $\underline{380}$, 19-27

BERNE, R. M. /1963/ Cardiac nucleotides in hypoxia: possible role in regulation of coronary blood flow. Am. J. Physiol. $\underline{204}$, 317-322

BERNE R. M. and RUBIO, R. /1974/ Adenine nucleotide metabolism in the heart. Circulat. Res. $\underline{34-35}$, III-109-120

BLAUSTEIN, M. P. /1979/ The role of calcium in catecholamine release from adrenergic nerve terminals. In: The Release of Catecholamines from Adrenergic Neurons /ed. by Paton, D. M./, Pergamon Press, Oxford, pp. 39-58

BLINKS, J. R. /1966/ Field stimulation as a means of effecting the graded release of autonomic transmitters in isolated heart muscle. J. Pharmacol. exp. Ther. $\underline{151}$, 221-235

BURNSTOCK, G. /1972/ Purinergic nerves. Pharmacol. Rev. $\underline{24}$, 509-581

BURNSTOCK, G. /1976/ Purinergic receptors. J. theor. Biol. $\underline{62}$, 491-503

BURNSTOCK, G. /1978/ A basis for distinquishing two types of purinergic receptor. In: Cell Membrane Receptors for Drugs and Hormones: A Multidisciplinary Approach /Straub, R. W. and Bolis, L. eds/, Raven Press, New York, pp. 107-118

BURNSTOCK, G. /1980/ Purinergic receptors in the heart.
Circulat. Res. __46__, I-175-182

CLANACHAN, A. S., JOHNS, A. and PATON, D. M. /1977/ Presynaptic
inhibitory actions of adenine nucleotides and adenosine on
neurotransmission in rat vas deferens. Neuroscience. __2__,
597-602

CLARENBACH, P., RAFFEL, G., MEYER, D. K. and HERTTING, G. /1976/
Inhibition by indomethacin and niflumic acid of catechol-
amine-uptake into rat hypothalamic and striatal synapto-
somes. Arch. int. Pharmacodyn. __219__, 79-86

DEGENRING, F. H., RUBIO, R. and BERNE, R. M. /1975/ Adenine
nucleotide metabolism during cardiac hypertrophy and
ischaemia in rats. J. mol. cell. Cardiol. __7__, 105-113

ENERO, M. A. and SAIDMAN, B. Q. /1977/ Possible feed-back inhibition of noradrenaline release by purine compounds.
Naunyn-Schmiedeberg's Arch. Pharmacol. __297__, 39-46

FRAME, M. H. and HEDQUIST, P. /1975/ Evidence for prostaglandin
mediated prejunctional control of renal sympathetic transmitter release and vascular tone. Br. J. Pharmacol. __54__,
189-196

HADHÁZY, P. and NÁDOR, T. /1976/ Effects of indomethacin and
PGE_1 on the vasoconstrictor responses of the rabbit ear
artery to nerve stimulation. Prostaglandins. __11__, 241-250

HADHÁZY, P., VIZI, E. S., MAGYAR, K. and KNOLL, J. /1976/
Inhibition of adrenergic neurotransmission by prostaglandin E_1 /PGE_1/ in the rabbit ear artery. Neuropharmacology.
__15__, 245-250

HEDQUIST, P. /1974/ Prostaglandin action on noradrenaline release and mechanical responses in the stimulated guinea
pig vas deferens. Acta Physiol. Scand. __90__, 86-93

HEDQUIST, P. and FREDHOLM, B. B. /1976/ Effects of adenosine on
adrenergic transmission; prejunctional inhibition and post-
junctional enhancement. Naunyn-Schmiedeberg's Arch.
Pharmacol. __293__, 217-223

HEDQUIST, P. and FREDHOLM, B. B. /1979/ Inhibitory effect of adenosine on adrenergic neuroeffector transmission in the rabbit heart. Acta Physiol. Scand. <u>105</u>, 120-122

HERLIHY, J. T., BOCKMAN, E. L., BERNE, R. M. and RUBIO, R. /1976/ Adenosine relaxation of isolated vascular smooth muscle. Am J. Physiol. <u>230</u>, 1239-1243

ILLÉS, P., HADHÁZY, P., TORMA, Z., VIZI, E. S. and KNOLL, J. /1973/ The effect of number of stimuli and rate of stimulation on the inhibition by PGE_1 of adrenergic transmission. Eur. J. Pharmacol. <u>24</u>, 29-36

JUHÁSZ-NAGY, A., GRÓSZ, G. and SZABÓ, Z. /1979/ "Purinergic" modulation of cardiac sympathetic activity. Abstracts Book of Cardiology Meeting, Balatonfüred, pp. 53-54 /in Hung./

KHAN, M. T. and MALIK, K. U. /1980/ Inhibitory effect of adenosine and adenine nucleotides on potassium-evoked efflux of /^{3}H/-noradrenaline from the rat isolated heart: lack of relationship to prostaglandins. Br. J. Pharmacol. <u>68</u>, 551-562

KNOLL, J., ILLÉS, P. and TORMA, Z. /1975/ The effect of PGE_2 on contraction delay and velocity of the field stimulated guinea-pig vas deferens. Neuropharmacol. <u>14</u>, 314-324

KOLASSA, N., PFLEGER, K. and RUMMEL, W. /1970/ Specificity of adenosine uptake into the heart and inhibition by dipyridamole. Eur. J. Pharmacol. <u>9</u>, 265-268

KÜBLER, W., SPIECKERMANN, P. G. and BRETSCHNEIDER, H. J. /1970/ Influence of dipyridamole /Persantin/ on myocardial adenosine metabolism. J. mol. cell Cardiol. <u>1</u>, 23-28

LANGER, S. Z., DUBOCOVICH, M. L. and CELUCH, S. M. /1975/ Prejunctional regulatory mechanisms for noradrenaline release elicited by nerve stimulation. In: <u>Chemical Tools in Catecholamine Research, Vol. II</u> /Almgren, C., Carlsson, A. and Engel, J. eds./ Elsevier, North Holland/USA, Amsterdam, pp. 183-191

LOKHANDWALA, M. F. /1979a/ Inhibition of cardiac sympathetic
neurotransmission by adenosine. Eur. J. Pharmacol.
60, 353-357

LOKHANDWALA, M. F. /1979b/ Presynaptic receptor systems on
cardiac sympathetic nerves. Life Sciences 24, 1823-1832

MUELLER, A. L., MOSIMANN, W. F. and WEINER, N. /1979/ Effects of
adenosine on neurally mediated norepinephrine release
from the cat spleen. Eur. J. Pharmacol. 53, 329-333

MULLER, M. J. and PATON, D. M. /1979/ Presynaptic inhibitory
actions of 2-substituted adenosine derivatives on neurotransmission in rat vas deferens: Effects of inhibitors
of adenosine uptake and deamination. Naunyn-Schmiedeberg's
Arch. Pharmacol. 306, 23-28

NEEDLEMAN, P., MINKES, M. S. and DOUGLAS, J. R. /1974/ Stimulation of prostaglandin biosynthesis by adenine nucleotides. Circulat. Res. 34, 455-460

NORTHOVER, B. J. /1971/ Mechanism of inhibitory action of indomethacin on smooth muscle. Br. J. Pharmacol. 41, 540-546

OLSSON, R. A. /1970/ Changes in content of purine nucleoside
in canine myocardium during coronary occlusion.
Circulat. Res. 26, 301-306

OLSSON, R. A., GENTRY, M. K. and SNOW, J. A. /1973/ Steric
requirements for binding of adenosine to a membrane carrier in canine heart. Biochim. Biophys. Acta 311, 242-250

OLSSON, R. A., SNOW, J. A., GENTRY, M. K. and FRICK, G. P.
/1972/ Adenosine uptake by canine heart. Circulat. Res.
31, 767-778

PATON, D. M. /1979a/ The Release of Catecholamines from Adrenergic Neurons. /ed. by D. M. Paton/ Pergamon Press, Oxford

PATON, D. M. /1979b/ Presynaptic inhibition of adrenergic
neurotransmission by adenine nucleotides and adenosine
In: Physiological and Regulatory Functions of Adenosine
and Adenine Nucleotides /Baer, H.P. and Drummond, G. I.
eds./ Raven Press, New York, pp. 69-77

RUBIO, R. and BERNE, R. M. /1969/ Release of adenosine by the normal myocardium in dogs and its relationship to the regulation of coronary resistence. Circulat. Res. 25, 407-415

SCHRADER, J., BERNE, R. M. and RUBIO, R. /1972/ Uptake and metabolism of adenosine by human erythrocyte ghosts. Am. J. Physiol. 223, 159-166

SCHRADER, J., RUBIO, R. and BERNE, R. M. /1975/ Inhibition of slow action potentials of guinea pig atrial muscle by adenosine: a possible effect on Ca^{2+}-influx. J. mol. cell. Cardiol. 7, 427-433

STARKE, K., ENDO, T. and TAUBE, H. D. /1975/ Relative pre- and postsynaptic potencies of alfa-adrenoceptor agonists in the rabbit pulmonary artery. Naunyn-Schmiedeberg's Arch. Pharmacol. 291, 55-78

STARKE, K., TAUBE, M. D. and BOROWSKI, E. /1977/ Presynaptic receptor systems in catecholaminergic transmission. Biochem. Pharmacol. 26, 259-268

STJÄRNE, L. /1979/ Role of prostaglandins and cyclic adenosine monophate in release. In: The Release of Catecholamines from Adrenergic Neurons /ed. by D. M. Paton/, Pergamon Press, Oxford, pp. 111-142

SZENTMIKLÓSI, A. J., CSEPPENTŐ, Á. and SZEGI, J. /1979/ Effect of adenosine on the adrenergic neurotransmission of ventricular myocardium. Abstracts Book of 45th Meeting of Hungarian Physiological Society, Szeged, p. 235 /in Hung./

THOMAS, R. A., RUBIO, R. and BERNE, R. M. /1975/ Comparison of the adenine nucleotide metabolism of dog atrial and ventricular myocardium. J. mol. cell Cardiol. 7, 115-123

VERHAEGHE, R. H., VANHOUTTE, P. M. and SHEPHERD, J. T. /1977/ Inhibition of sympathetic neurotransmission in canine blood vessels by adenosine and adenine nucleotides. Circulat. Res. 40, 208-215

VIZI, E. S., SOMOGYI, G. T., HADHÁZY, P. and KNOLL, J. /1973/
Effect of duration and frequency of stimulation on the
presynaptic inhibition by alfa-adrenoceptor stimulation
of the adrenergic transmission.
Naunyn-Schmiedeberg's Arch. Pharmacol. $\underline{280}$, 79-91

WESTFALL, T. C. /1977/ Local regulation of adrenergic neurotransmission. Physiol. Rev. $\underline{57}$, 659-728

WESTFALL, T. C. and LEIGHTON, H. J. /1976/ Effect of decentral-
ization on presynaptic receptor regulation of NE release.
Pharmacologist. $\underline{18}$, 208

ZEHL, U., RITTER, C. and FÖRSTER, W. /1976/ Influence of prostaglandins upon adenosine release and of adenosine upon
prostaglandin release in the isolated rabbit heart.
Acta. Biol. Med. Germ. $\underline{35}$, K77-K82

Discussion

Kunos: Your results very convincingly show the inhibitory effect of adenosine on noradrenaline release. What do you think about the physiological role of this system compared to other ones that can produce "presynaptic" inhibition of release? /such as presynaptic alpha, opiate, muscarinic, etc./

Szentmiklosi: Berne and his associated have found that adenosine levels in hypoxic myocardium can rise to about 100 μmol/l. This concentration of adenosine was capable of inducing a nearly half-maximal suppression in the adrenergic neurotransmission of the ventricular myocardium. Therefore, adenosine released under ischaemic conditions might be contributed to the inhibition of adrenergic neurotransmission. Quite recently, Burnstock have found evidence for the existence of purinergic innervation of the heart muscle, too. This fact would be very important in respect of prejunctional regulation. I think, a critical question is, how the effects of exogenous and endogenous adenosine are comparable. Therefore, it would be too early to estabilish the participation of purinergic mechanisms compared to that of other presynaptic receptor structures.

Matthson: Does the concentration of adenosine in the heart under normal physiological conditions differ from that in other tissues?

Szentmiklosi: As far as I know, the adenosine concentration of different tissues has been of the same order of magnitude as that found in myocardium under physiological conditions. This means a μmolar concentration range.

Rubányi: Since extracellular Ca^{2+} exerts a membrane stabilizing effect when presents in high concentrations. The hypothesis, that adenosine inhibits Ca^{2+} influx should be studied more specifically by Ca^{2+}-antagonists.

Szentmiklosi: The question you have raised is an interesting aspect when explaining the results concerning the relation between adenosine and extracellular calcium. I agree with you, that the adenosine action should also be studied using specific calcium-antagonists. We have no experience in this respect, but Dr. Juhász-Nagy have reported last year, that the presence of specific antagonists of calcium channels were capable of preventing the coronary dilator action of adenosine. In the light of this important finding the molecular mechanisms of adenosine action might be approached more profoundly.

MODULATION BY ADENOSINE OF SYMPATHETIC RESPONSES IN THE IN SITU CANINE HEART

A. Juhász-Nagy

National Institute of Vascular Surgery, Semmelweis University Medical School, Budapest, Hungary

In the past few years a variety of mechanisms has been identified as modulators of adrenergic regulation of cardiac activity. This modulating action is a very extensive topic and only a selected aspect of it will be considered in the present paper. The principal attention will be directed toward the modulatory effect of adenine nucleosides, namely adenosine, on the three most important variables influenced by sympathetic activity: cardiac inotropism, frequency of heart beat and coronary blood flow. It has been recognized for over fifty years that adenosine, AMP, ADP, and ATP exert powerful vasodilatory action and induce bradycardia (Drury and Szent-Györgyi, 1929). The nucleotide compounds cannot readily cross cell membranes, but adenosine and its derivative inosine diffuse freely into the extracellular space. Even under resting conditions these substances are constantly formed by the heart and their release is enormously potentiated in response to a negative oxygen balance of the myocardium resulting in decreases of the energy charge of cardiac adenine nucleotide pools (Atkinson, 1968). In the past twenty years outstanding experimental analyses, especially the investigations of Berne and his co-workers (see Rubio and Berne, 1975), have provided evidence for the theory that adenosine plays a crucial role in the process by which the myocardium of warm blooded animals meets either hypoxic challange or increased work load. It is generally thought that periarterial accumulation of adenosine is the key mechanism that accounts for metabolic autoregulation (vasodilation) of the coronary vessels.

At the same time, it is only partially understood how the latter type of regulation is related to the adrenergic control of the _in situ_ heart; in many organs of the body the modulatory effect of "purinergic" mediators on adrenergic mechanisms is well documented (Moylan and Westfall, 1979; Burnstock, 1980).

Methods

Mongrel dogs varying in weight from 14 to 22 kg were narcotized with pentobarbital sodium (30 to 35 mg/kg i.v.). Supplementary doses were administered as needed. The trachea was intubated and positive pressure ventilation with room air was started immediately after anaesthesia. The chest was opened bilaterally in the fourth intercostal space and the pericardium was slit to expose the heart. In order to measure myocardial contractile force Walton-Brodie strain gauge arches were sewn to the anterior apex and the lateral base of the left ventricle. A third gauge was sutured to the right ventricular base. The myocardial segment between the two feet of the gauges was stretched by about 30 percent of its initial length to ensure the relative independence of the measured force from ventricular geometry and performance.

In another series of experiments a short segment of the left anterior desecending (LAD) coronary artery, close to its origin, was dissected free and a Statham electromagnetic flow probe of appropriate size (usually 2 mm) was placed around the vessel. The probe was connected to a Statham SP 2202 electromagnetic flowmeter. Phasic as well as mean coronary blood flows were measured, the latter value being obtained by electrical integration. Aortic pressure was recorded with the aid of a Statham trancducer (P 23AA) connected to a polyethylene catheter introduced through the femoral artery. Heart rate was computed from pressure tracings. All recordings were made on a six-channel Hellige recorder.

The left stellate ganglion was exposed in each experiment and a bipolar platinum electrode was positioned on the anterior ansa subclavia for the duration of the investigation. The ansa was stimulated by 30 second trains of rectangular pulses of 6-8 V, 3 msec duration at frequencies of 1, 2, 4, 8 and 20 Hz, respectively. After recording the control responses, the same maneuvers were repeated during adenosine infusions. The drug was administered in increasing doses of 0.008, 0.031, 0.125, and 0.25 mg/kg/min, each dose infused for a period of time suitable for the examination of the consequences of adenosine on the effects of sympathetic stimulation. The drug was infused directly into the left heart, in order to prevent, as far as possible, uptake and enzymatic degradation. For this purpose a polyethylene cannula was inserted through the left auricular appendage.

Circulatory variables were chosen for data analysis during steady state values of control periods and during near steady state values at the terminal periods of stimulations. Inotropic responses were characterized as percentage changes, heart rate responses as beat/min, whereas the coronary response was expressed as a calculated mean vascular resistance (pressure/flow). All values quoted in the text are means ± S.E. The results were examined statistically using the Student's t test for paired data.

Results

Inotropic responses

Fig. 1. illustrates the experimental protocol and depicts the modulatory effect of adenosine on ventricular contractile responses induced by sympathetic stimulation. In the first (control) block of the figure the dependence of inotropic responses on stimulus frequencies could readily be observed, together with the variability of responses in the different regions of the heart: the effects are greatest in the left ventricular base and smallest in the apex. Irrespective of this variability, however, the responses were found to be reduced by adenosine administration, especially at lower stimulus frequencies. At the largest adenosine dose employed (last block of Fig. 1.), only the contractility increase induced by the maximum frequency is conspicuous. Statistical analysis of the responses is given in Fig. 2. Considering

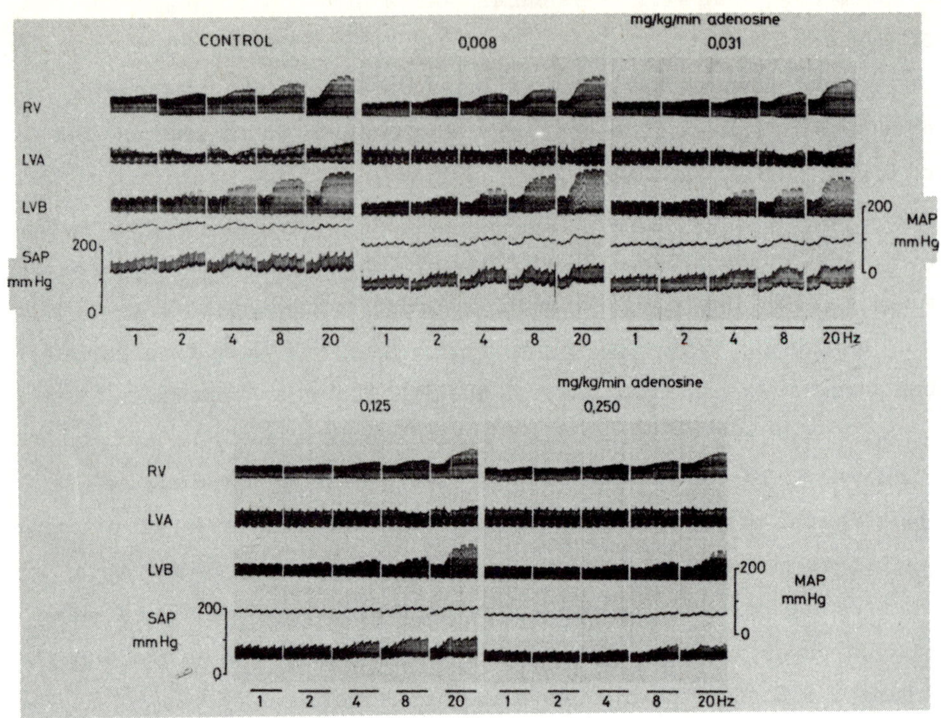

Fig. 1. Modulatory effect of adenosine infusions on inotropic responses induced by sympathetic stimulation. From above downwards in each block: myocardial contractile force (strain gauge) measured in the right ventricle (RV), left ventricular apex (LVA), and left ventricular base (LVB), mean arterial blood pressure (MAP), systemic arterial pressure (SAP). Horizontal bars below records denote stimulation periods of 30 sec duration.

the topographic inhomogenity of sympathetically-induced local inotropic effects, a fact well known from data reported by Szentiványi and his co-workers (Szentiványi et al., 1967; Randall et al., 1968), percent contractility increases from the three regions were averaged in computing the changes at any single event of the pattern. At the same time, it is apparent from this pattern that the adenosine-induced inhibition of the inotropic effects is directly proportional to the dose of the nucleoside and inversely proportional to the stimulus frequency. This twofold interaction is visualized in the three dimensional diagram of Fig. 3. by plotting sympathetic contractile responses simultaneously

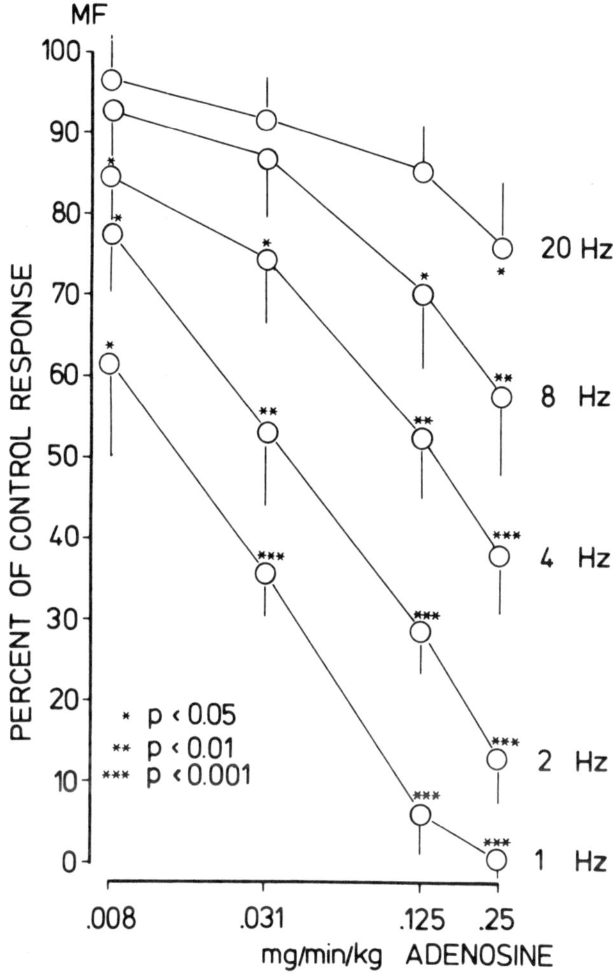

Fig. 2. Inhibition of sympathetic inotropic responses by adenosine. Mean values ± S.E. of eight experiments. MF myocardial contractile force. Hz frequency of stimulation.

against the two independent variables: adenosine dose and stimulus frequency.

Chronotropic responses

In contrast to the fact that only slight decreases of resting ventricular contractility could be detected in hearts subjected to adenosine infusions up to 0.25 mg/kg/min (note the almost horizontal

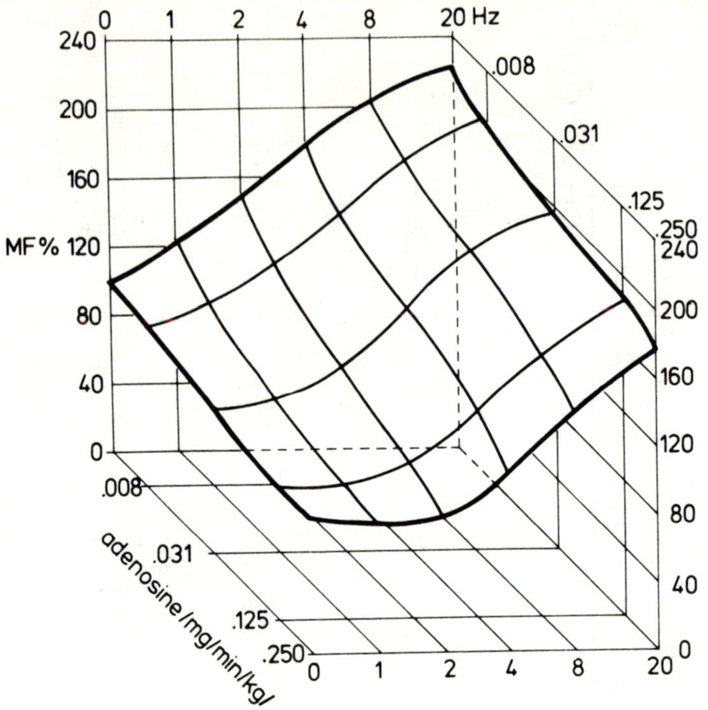

Fig. 3. The change in myocardial contractile force (MF) as a function of the frequency of supramaximal sympathetic stimulation and the dose of adenosine infusion. The response surface represents the mean data from eight dogs.

position of the left edge of response surface in Fig. 3.), heart rate is considerably affected by adenosine even under resting conditions (Fig. 4.). Otherwise, the adenosine-induced inhibition of sympathetic chronotropic responses seems to be very similar to that observed in inotropism. Again, by comparing the anterior and posterior opposing edges of the response surface, it is apparent that a progressive increase in the frequency of sympathetic stimulation produces responses which are more resistant to adenosine-inhibition than responses elicited at lower frequencies of stimulation.

Coronary responses

The response surface illustrated in Fig. 5. presents a more

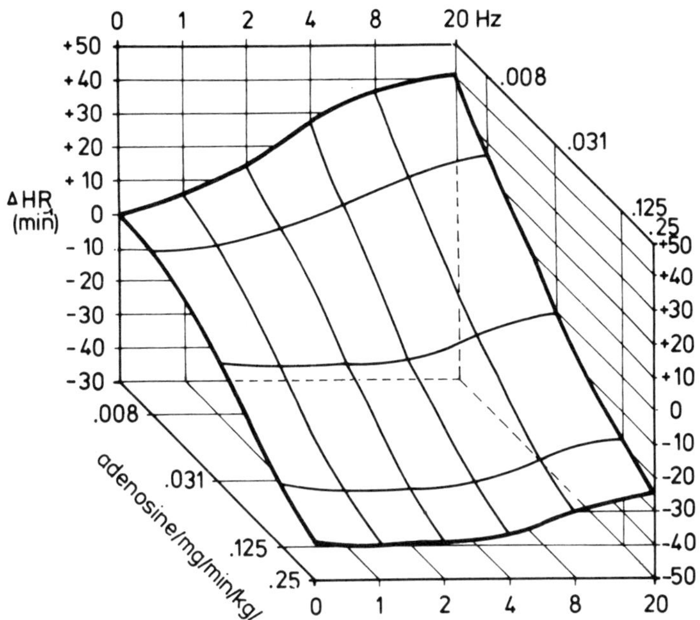

Fig. 4. The change of heart rate (HR) as a function of the frequency of supramaximal sympathetic stimulation and the dose of adenosine infusion. Mean data from eight dogs.

complicated landscape than the former ones. In contrast with inotropism, and similarly to chronotropism, adenosine exerts a powerful
influence on coronary vascular resistance. So does sympathetic stimulation. However, the interaction of these two vasodilator mechanisms is
more equivocal than the interaction seen in former figures. The flattened lower edge of the response surface is a dramatic expression of
the insensitivity of maximally dilated vessels to an additional adrenergic stimulus. This absence of sympathetic vasodilation of beta-type
could equally be ascribed to inhibitory interactions, to secondary hemodynamic causes, or both. The inspection of the diagram reveals another
type of interaction, i.e. reversal of the vasodilator sympathetic
effect. These vasoconstrictor responses appear as "humps" on the
response surface, and they are characteristic of common ordinates related to moderate adenosine doses and submaximal sympathetic stimulus

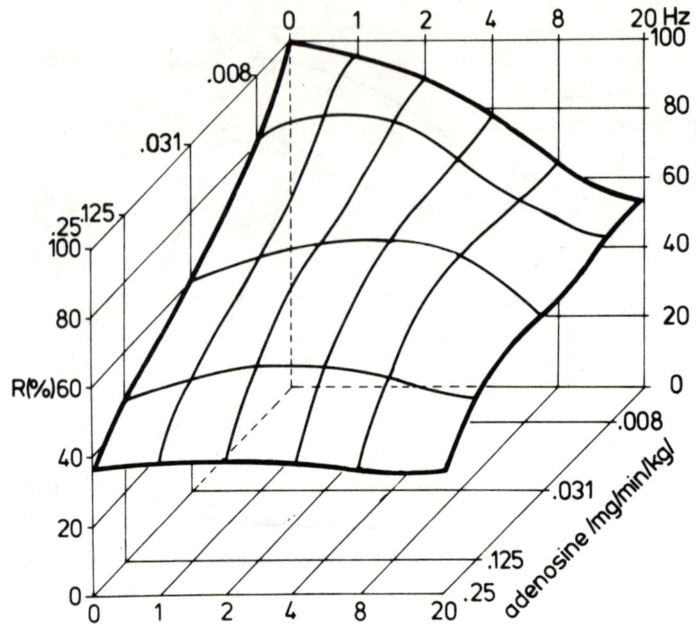

Fig. 5. The change of calculated mean vascular coronary resistance (R) as a function of the frequency of supramaximal
sympathetic stimulation and the dose of adenosine infusion.
Mean data from eight dogs.

frequencies. An example is given in Fig. 6. The fact that the increase
of calculated vascular resistance could also be observed in the end-
diastolic phase of flow when the vessels are free of extravascular
compression exerted by the ventricular muscle (see Fig. 6.), proves
the true vasomotor character of the constrictor response.

Discussion

The negative inotropic effect of adenosine on atrial muscle is a
well established fact (Hollander and Webb, 1957; de Gubareff and
Sleator, 1965; Schrader et al., 1975; Szentmiklósi et al., 1976).
Since, as it has been shown by Szentmiklósi et al. (1976) this action
is antagonized competetively by methylxanthines, adenosine apparently
affects P_1 "purinoceptors" (see Burnstock, 1980) located in the atrial

92

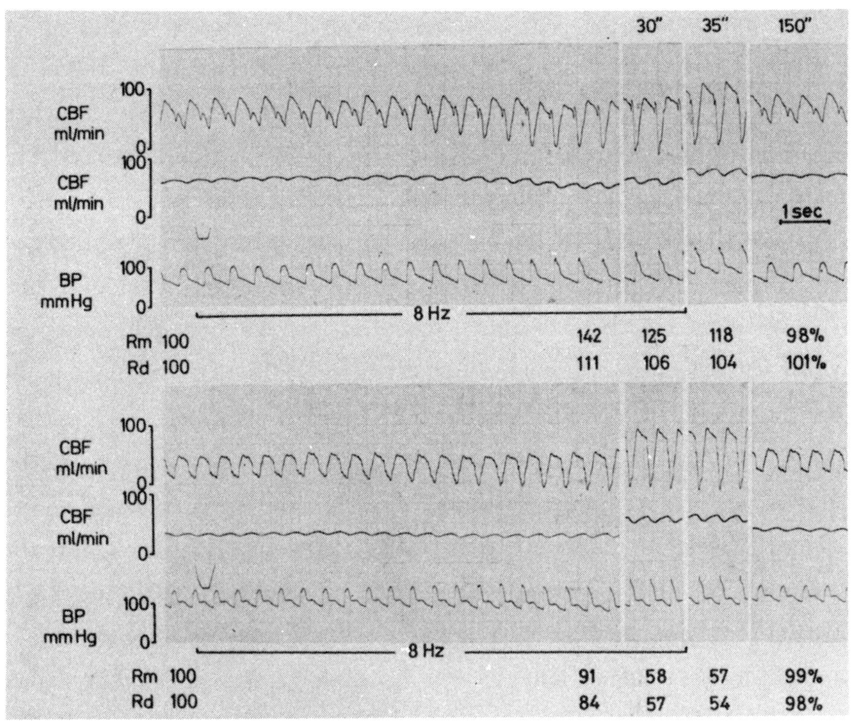

Fig. 6. Comparison of coronary effects of left ansa stimulation obtained in the control state (lower panels) and during the infusion of 0.031 mg/kg/min adenosine (upper panels). Representative tracings taken at high paper speed. From above downwards: phasic and mean coronary blood flow (CBF), arterial blood pressure (BP). Signs above the pressure curve denote the beginning of the stimulation. Rm and Rd: mean and end-diastolic coronary vascular resistance.

region of the heart. Similarly, the nucleoside has a negative chronotropic effect of its own (Drury and Szent-Györgyi, 1929; Johnson and McKinnon, 1956; James 1965) associated with a blockade of Ca^{2+} influx through the slow channels of the cell membrane (Schrader et al., 1975). By contrast, no change of ventricular inotropism could be detected in isolated (Wedd, 1931; Drury, 1932) and in situ (Lammerant and Becsei, 1973) heart preparations subjected to high doses of adenosine.

The results of the present experiments show that although the effect of adenosine on basal (resting) ventricular contractility is very slight, the compound can affect considerably the contractile force in ventricular muscle influenced by an augmented sympathetic drive. The experiments were undertaken to determine if adenosine has the capacity to reduce the enhancement of cardiac excitation (and metabolism) induced by adrenergic nerve fibres, and to explore the possible role of this putative interaction in the physiologic and pathologic regulation of cardiac activity. According to the results obtained the first question could be answered affirmatively. Regarding the second question, i.e. the extent to which this interaction is responsible for modulating the cardiostimulatory adrenergic responses under physiologic and pathologic circumstances, it can only be resolved by further studies. It is known that adenosine is constantly released even by the well oxygenated myocardial cells. Under these circumstances, however, the concentration of the compound in the extracellular fluid is probably very low (less than 1 nM/g of tissue, Rubio and Berne, 1969). At the same time, concomitant with a reduction of oxygen delivery (Berne, 1963) or an increased oxygen need (Foley _et al._, 1978), the formation of adenosine significantly increases. The same happens, according to recent findings during the stimulation of cardiac efferent sympathetic fibres (Miller et al., 1979).

The lowest dose of exogenous adenosine employed in the present study (0.008 mg/kg/min) corresponds, according to our former experiments (Juhász-Nagy and Nemes, 1980), to the threshold dose with intrauricular administration, whereas the higher doses (0.125 - 0.25 mg/kg/min) correspond to the upper, flattened portion of the adenosine dose response curve. It is possible, therefore, that the modulatory influence observed in the present experiments covers the whole range of the negative feedback effect of adenosine on adrenergic regulation. On the other hand, considering the possible differences in action of endogenously released and exogenously administered compounds, too bold speculations along these lines are unwarranted until more information becomes available concerning the transport characteristics and extracellular   fluid composition of cardiac tissue.

Both alpha and beta adrenoceptors are known to exist in the heart muscle and coronary vessels. Unlike the similar (although not equipotent) role played by them in the myocardium, alpha and beta adrenoceptor stimulation elicit diametrically opposite effects in the coronary vessel wall. The net vasodilator effects observed under physiologic conditions on sympathetic stimulation indicate the preponderance of the beta action over the alpha. This unequivocal predominance of the beta vasodilator effects seems to be lessened under the influence of adenosine. In some cases, even the unmasking of the alpha-constrictor action was observed (Fig. 6.). It is tempting to speculate that the increased percentage of alpha-coronary vasoconstrictor influence in hearts subjected to temporary myocardial ischaemia (Aviado and Juhász-Nagy, this symposium) is related to the effect of the myocardial "hypoxic-transmitter" adenosine.

Summary

Adenosine infused into the left atrium of narcotized, open chest dogs was found to modulate, in a dose-dependent manner, sympathetic excitatory responses induced by electrical stimulation of cardiac adrenergic fibres. Adenosine inhibited the positive inotropic and chronotropic effects and unmasked, in some cases, vasoconstrictor adrenergic influences on coronary flow.

References

Atkinson, D. E.: Energy charge of the adenylate pool as a regulatory parameter: interaction with feedback modifiers. Biochemistry, 7: 4030-4034, 1968.

Berne, R. M.: Cardiac nucleotides in hypoxia: possible role in regulation of coronary blood flow. Am. J. Physiol. 204: 317-322, 1963.

Burnstock, G.: Purinergic receptors in the heart. Circ. Res. 46: I-175-I-182/suppl./, 1980.

de Gubareff, T. and Sleator, W.: Effect of caffeine on mammalian
atrial muscle, and its interaction with adenosine and calcium. J.
Pharmacol. exp. Ther. 148: 202-214, 1965.

Drury, A. N.: Nucleic acid derivatives and the heart beat. J. Physiol.
(Lond.) 74: 147-155, 1932.

Drury, A. N. and Szent-Györgyi, A.: The physiological activity of
adenine compounds with especial reference to their action upon the
mammalian heart. J. Physiol. (Lond.) 68: 213-237, 1929.

Foley, D. H.; Herlihy, J.T., Thompson, C. I., Rubio, R. and Berne,
R. M.: Increased adenosine formation by rat myocardium with acute
aortic constriction. J. mol. cell. Cardiol. 10: 293-300, 1978.

Hollander, P. B. and Webb, J. L.: Effects of adenine nucleotides on
the contractility and membrane potentials of rat atrium. Circ. Res.
5: 349-353, 1957.

James, T. N.: The chronotropic action of ATP and related compounds
studied by direct perfusion of sinus node. J. Pharmacol. exp.Ther.
149: 233-247, 1965.

Johnson, E. A. and McKinnon, M. G.: Effect of acetylcholine and
adenosine on cardiac cellular potentials. Nature, 178: 1174-1175,
1956.

Juhász-Nagy, A. and Nemes, A.: Verapamil inhibits reactive hyperemia
and adenosine-induced vasodilation in the canine coronary bed. in
press., 1980.

Lammerant, J. and Becsei, I.: Left ventricular contractility and
developed tension in the intact dog submitted to an intracoronary
infusion of adenosine. J. Physiol. (Lond.) 229 : 41-49, 1973.

Miller, W. L., Belardinelli, L., Bacchus, A., Foley, D. H., Rubio,
R. and Berne, R. M.: Canine myocardial adenosine and lactate production, oxygen consumption, and coronary blood flow during
stellate ganglia stimulation. Circ. Res. 45: 708-718, 1979.

Moylan, R. D. and Westfall, T. C.: Effect of adenosine and adrenergic neurotransmission in the superfused rat portal vein. Blood
Vessels 16 : 302-310, 1979.

Randall, W. C., Szentiványi, M., Pace, J. B., Wechsler, J. S. and
Kaye, M. P.: Patterns of sympathetic nerve projections onto the
canine heart. Circ. Res. 22 : 315-323, 1968.

Rubio, R. and Berne, R. M.: Release of adenosine by the normal myocardium in dogs and its relationship to the regulation of coronary
resistance. Circ. Res. _25_: 407-415, 1969.

Rubio, R. and Berne, R. M.: Regulation of coronary blood flow. Progr.
Cardiovasc. Dis. _18_: 105-122, 1975.

Schrader, J., Rubio, R. and Berne, R. M.: Inhibition of slow action
potentials of guinea-pig atrial muscle by adenosine: A possible effect
of Ca^{2+} influx. J. mol. cell. Cardiol. _7_: 427-433, 1975.

Szentiványi, M., Pace, J. P., Wechsler, J. S. and Randall, W. C.:
Localized myocardial responses to stimulation of cardiac sympathetic nerves. Circ. Res. _21_: 691-702, 1967.

Szentmiklósi, J., Takács, I. and Szegi, J.: Studies on the inotropic
and chronotropic effects of adenosine. In: Szekeres, L. and Papp,
J. Gy. (eds.): Symposium on Pharmacology of the heart. pp. 81-86,
Akadémiai Kiadó, Budapest, 1976.

Wedd, A. M.: The action of adenosine and certain related compounds
on coronary flow of the perfused heart of the rabbit. J. Pharmacol.
exp. Ther. _41_: 355-366, 1931.

<u>Discussion</u>

<u>Kunos</u>: Your presentation was exemplary not only in its contents
but also in its format. The last of your three-dimensional
figures revealed that, under certain experimental conditions,
adenosine may enhance the alpha-adrenergic coronary vasoconstrictor effect of sympathetic stimulation. This may involve
mechanisms other than inhibition of catecholamine release.

<u>Juhász-Nagy</u>: From the hemodynamic point of view the most obvi-
ous explanation is that adenosine by enhancing coronary blood
flow and by decreasing coronary arteriovenous oxygen difference as well, creates conditions for the heart to encounter
the augmented O_2 demand due to adrenergic excitation in the
simplest way: to increase O_2 extraction instead of flow increase. The alpha-adrenoceptors of the coronary vessels could,
therefore, exert an unopposed vasoconstrictor action. The
alpha-stimulation cannot do that under ordinary circumstances
because of the maximal, or nearly maximal O_2 extraction effected by the resting myocardium. Accordingly, vasodilation of
any type, provided it is accompanied by the decrease of cardiac
O_2 demand, favours a <u>priori</u> the alpha-component of any subsequent adrenergic stimulus. It should be remembered that similar
things happen when sympathetic stimulation is superimposed on
vagal stimulation as it was shown many years ago by Dr. Szentiványi and yourself. However, it is not difficult to interpret
the appearance of alpha-vasoconstriction during adenosine effect in terms of a more specific reciprocal interaction between
alpha- and beta-adrenoceptors and adenosine, respectively.

<u>Kunos</u>: It has recently been described by Stouffer et al. that
in hypothyroid rats beta-mediated lipolysis is decreased and
the alpha-mediated lipolysis is increased in fat cells. This
change is reversed by <u>in vitro</u> addition of adenosine deaminase
to suspensions of adipocytes from hypothyroid rats.
Did you investigate adenosine deaminase effect in your experimental system?

<u>Juhász-Nagy</u>: Thank you for the interesting information about
adipocytes; adenosine could affect coronary adrenoceptors along
the same lines. My answer to your last question is: no. At the
same time, we know that the deaminated product of adenosine:
inosine, does not affect the adrenoceptors similarly to adenosine. In contrast to adenosine, it stimulates beta-adrenoceptors
rather than inhibits them. More interestingly, inosine can re-
activate cardiac and coronary beta-adrenoceptors blocked with
pharmacological agents such as propranolol. This is depicted
in the next figure. You can see that the effects of left stellate ganglion stimulation were partially blocked by propranolol /panel B/, then almost completely restored by inosine
/panel C/. Since there is clearly no signs that inosine liber-
ates catecholamines from the heart, and since the same restoration could be effected regarding the effects of exogenous
catecholamines, inosine apparently acts on the adrenoceptors

themselves.

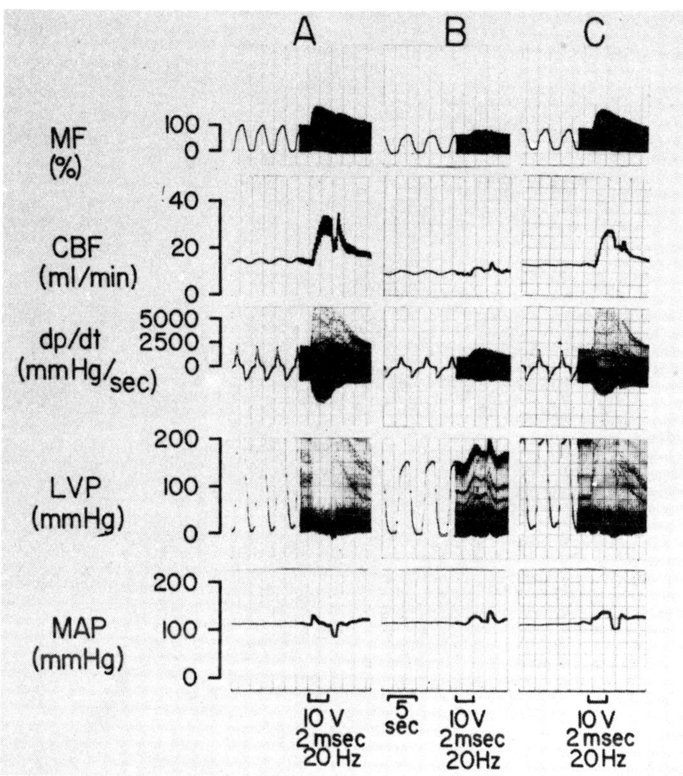

<u>Fig.</u> Experiment on open chest dog.
From above downwards: myocardial contractile force /strain gauge/, coronary blood flow in the LAD artery, dp/dt_{max} of left ventricular pressure, left ventricular pressure, mean arterial pressure.
Stellate stimulation as indicated. Between A and B 0.2 mg/kg propranolol was given intravenously; between B and C 5 mg/kg/min inosine was infunded i.v. for 10 min. Fifteen min elapsed between B and C.

RESTORATION BY INOSINE OF DESENSITIZED BETA-ADRENOCEPTORS IN THE CANINE CORONARY BED

L. Papp. Z. Szabó and A. Juhász-Nagy
National Institute of Vascular Surgery, Semmelweis University Medical School, Budapest, Hungary

Introduction

Prolonged exposure to large doses of adrenergic agonists leads
to a characteristic progressive decrease of the subsequent
adrenergic response. This phenomenon, termed tachyphylaxis, is
intimately related to the physiologic regulation of the adrenergic receptors. A plausible explanation for the attenuating
influence of the agonists on their own effect is a reversible
decrease of the active receptor number resulting from modulation of receptor affinity or receptor responsiveness, or both.
The phenomenon may be related either to the depletion or the
accumulation of some stimulatory or inhibitory modulating
substances, respectively.

Formerly, it has been reported that inosine, a common breakdown product of the adenine nucleotide metabolism in the body,
is able to restore in the in situ canine heart the responsiveness of cardiac /coronary/ beta-adrenoceptors partially
blocked with propranolol /Juhász-Nagy and Aviado, 1977./.
The present study describes the reversal by inosine of the
beta-adrenergic action partially inactivated after exposure to
large doses of isoproterenol. Because of its great practical
importance in the sympathetic circulatory response, the
coronary beta-adrenergic effect was selected to characterize
the resensitizing process.

Methods

Mongrel dogs varying in weight from 12 kg to 19 kg were narcotized with penthobarbital sodium /30 to 35 mg/kg i.v./.
Supplementary doses were administered as needed. The trachea
was intubated and positive pressure ventilation with room air
was started immediately after anaesthesia. The chest was opened
in the fourth, left intercostal space.The animals were instrumented as described in the previous paper /Juhász-Nagy, this
symposium /.

Tachyphylaxic desensitization of the coronary beta-receptors
was established by i.v. infusion of isoproterenol /Isuprel,
Winthrop/. Isoproterenol was diluted in physiologic salt
solution to obtain a concentration /W/V/ of 1 /ug x kg b.w./
2.25 ml, and was delivered intravenously at a 2.25 ml/min rate.
The total infusion time varied from 20 to 30 minutes/v.i./.
Inosine /5 mg x kg b.w./ 9 ml/min/ was administered in the
same manner for 10 min. Coronary beta-receptor sensitivity
was challenged under steady state circulatory conditions: the
criterion used for this was the stabilization of systemic
blood pressure after the infusions of isoproterenol and inosine, respectively.

Two types of challenging procedures were employed in two different experimental groups.

I. Responses to sympathetic stimulation were measured in ten
experiments - designated as Experimental Group I - in which
the left stellate ganglion was exposed and a bipolar platinum
electrode was positioned on the left anterior ansa for the
duration of the experiment. The ansa was stimulated by 60
second trains of rectangular pulses of 8-10 V, 3 msec duration
at a freguency of 20 Hz. The electrical stimulation of the
ansa was performed at last twice before and after each of the
following infusions: inosine /5 mg/kg/min for 10 min/ - Sub-
group I/A - and isoproterenol /1 /ug/kg/min for 20 min/ and
a subsequent administration of inosine /5 mg/kg/min for 10
min/ - Sub-group I/B. The dose of isoproterenol used in the
latter experiments was the minimum required to produce a rep-
roducible tachyphylaxic change in the beta-receptor sensitivity. The sequence used in Sub-group A permitted an
examination of the consequences of inosine on the coronary
effects of sympathetic stimulation.

II. Another six experiments - designated as Experimental Group
II. - were performed under comparable conditions, except that
beta-receptor sensitivity was tested by i.v. administration
of the sympathetic transmitter noradrenaline, ranging from
0.125 to 2.0 /ug/kg to obtain a dose response relationship.
The administration of challenging noradrenaline doses was
repeated after infusion of isoproterenol /1 /ug/kg/min for
30 min/ and inosine /5 mg/kg/min for 10 min/, respectively.

Coronary reactions were characterized as mean flow recordings
as well as percent coronary vascular conductances. In Group I.
the magnitude of these reactions was defined by averaging
mean flow and mean coronary conductance changes determined
at 6 sec intervals during the 60 sec stimulation periods. In
II. the criterion of the dilatory response was maximum change
of coronary conductance.

Statistical analysis of the results were performed using the
Student's t-test for paired data. All values quoted in the
text are mean ± standard error.

Results

I. Sympathetic stimulation

A. Effect of inosine Basic hemodynamic values of coronary circulation, as shown in the Table I., exhibited moderate but statistically significant changes after inosine infusion. However, vasodilator responses induced by sympathetic stimulation were not considerably affected after the administration of the drug.

B. Effects of isoproterenol and inosine This group was pretreated with a large of isoproterenol and then subsequently received the same dose of inosine as the former group. Isoproterenol infusion elicited the well known coronary vasodilatation of beta type. After the infusion period was completed and the systemic blood pressure returned to its pre-infusion level/Table II./ the resting coronary vascular tone was still slightly below i.e. the percent value of coronary conductance slightly above the control level. This new equilibrium of coronary vascular tone was associated with a significantly diminished vasodilatory response to sympathetic stimulation. The typical example of the this tachyphylaxic decrease is depicted in Fig 1. On administration of inosine the sympathetic dilatory response returned to to the pre-tachyphylaxic state.

II. Noradrenaline administration

Coronary effects induced by challenging doses of noradrenaline were quantitatively,as well as qualitatively similar to those induced by neural stimulation. The tachyphylaxic decrease of beta-adrenergic sensitivity caused the coronary dose response curve of noradrenaline to make a shift to the right /Fig. 2./ without any appreciable change in the simultaneous pressor response of the drug /Fig. 3./. On administration of inosine coronary vasodilator responses returned to their control values. The latter drug also failed to affect the systemic pressor responses induced by noradrenaline. Similarly to the maximal responses used to construct the dose response curves, duration and course of the adrenergic coronary vasodilatory actions, as depicted in Fig. 4., exhibited the same characteristic behavior. Averaged vasodilator maxima obtained by with the latter type of calculation were found to be somewhat smaller than those shown in Fig. 2; this slight difference is due to the imperfect temporal coincidence of vasodilator peaks in the different animals.

Discussion

The effect of massive isoproterenol doses on the general circulatory responses of catecholamines in anaesthetized dogs and cats has been extensively studied by Walz and Maengwyn-Davies /1960/, Walz et al. /1960/, and Butterworth /1963/. The above mentioned authors described that the vasodepressor

103

Table I.

Sympathetic coronary responses of dogs treated with inosine[+]

	Mean arterial pressure /mmHg/		Mean LAD blood flow /ml min^{-1}/		Coronary conductance /%/	
	Pre-stim.	Change	Pre-stim.	Change	Pre-stim.	Change
Control	114 $\pm$ 10	+14 $\pm$ 3[a]	19.1 $\pm$ 2.5	+13.4 $\pm$2.9[a]	100 $\pm$ 0	+49 $\pm$ 4[a]
After inosine	107 $\pm$ 7	+11 $\pm$ 2[a]	22.5 $\pm$ 3.1[b]	+13.1 $\pm$ 3.0[a]	125 $\pm$ 5[b]	+53 $\pm$ 9[a]

+ Values are reported as mean $\pm$ S.E.M. /n=4/
a Significant change /p$<$0.05/ from pre-stimulus value
b Significant change /p$<$0.05/ from control value
LAD left anterior descending coronary artery

Table II.

Sympathetic coronary responses of dogs treated with isoproterenol and inosine[+]

	Mean arterial pressure /mmHg/		Mean LAD blood flow /ml min^{-1}/		Coronary conductance /%/	
	Pre-stim.	Change	Pre-stim.	Change	Pre-stim.	Change
Control	103 ± 2	+18 ± 3[a]	25.3 ± 4.6	+16.2 ± 2.1[a]	100 ± 0	+43 ± 8[a]
After isopro-terenol	108 ± 5	+16 ± 2[a]	32.8 ± 6.6[b]	+ 8.3 ± 2.2[ab]	124 ± 6[b]	+14 ± 7[b]
After inosine	107 ±11	+12 ± 5	33.5 ± 5.0[b]	+15.0 ± 2.0[a]	134 ± 6[b]	+46 ± 14[a]

+ Values are reported as mean ± S.E.M. /n=6/
a Significant change /p < 0.05/ from pre-stimulus value
b Significant change /p < 0.05/ from control value
LAD left anterior descending coronary artery

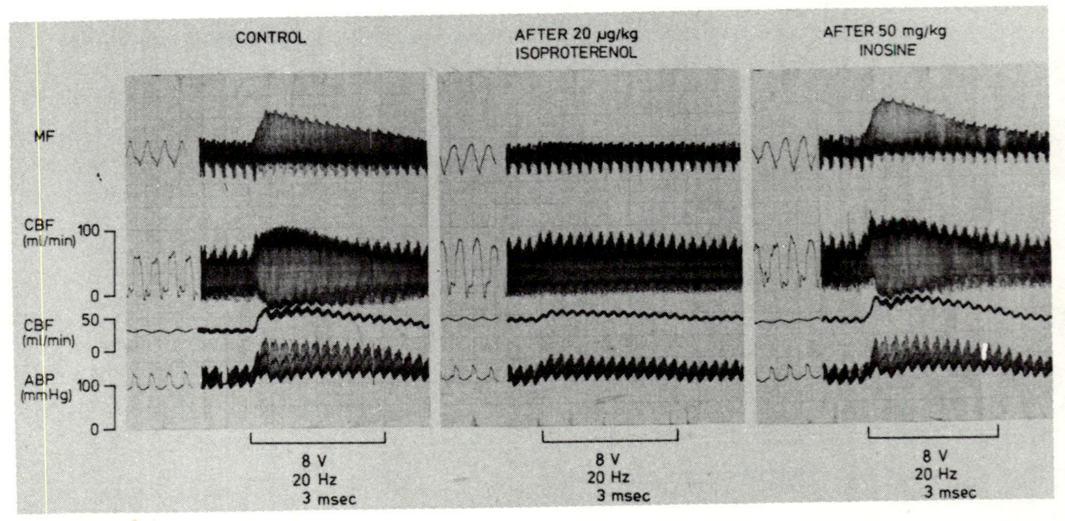

Fig. 1. Cardiovascular responses induced by sympathetic stimulation. From above downwards: myocardial contractile force /strain gauge/, phasic and mean coronary blood flow, arterial blood pressure.

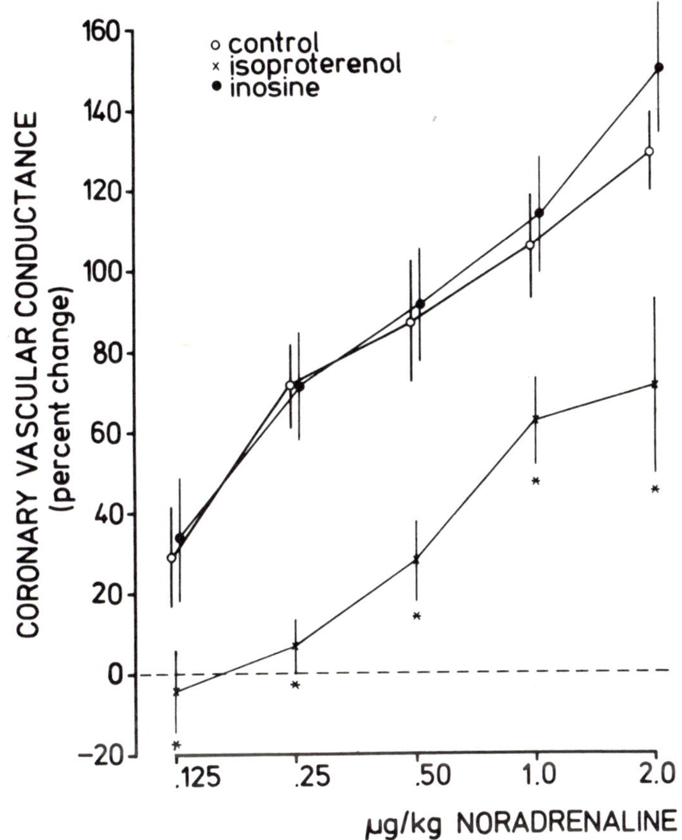

<u>Fig. 2.</u> Coronary dose response curves to noradrenaline.
Asterisks refer to significant changes /p<0.05/.
Mean values + S.E.
Infusion of isoproterenol in a massive dose
/30 µg/kg/ caused the dose response curve to make
a parallel shift to the right.
Infusion of inosine /50 mg/kg/ reshifted the curve
to the control state.
n=6

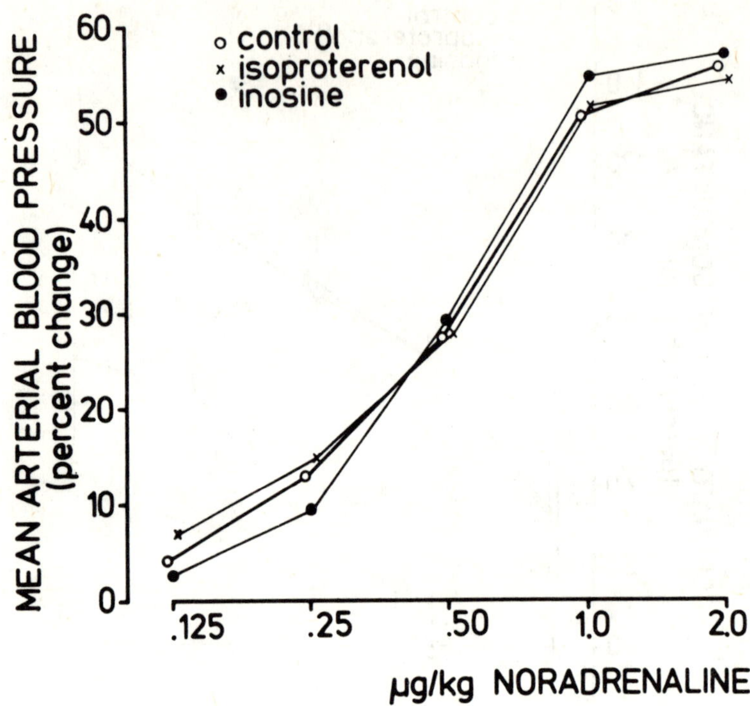

Fig. 3. Dose response curves of the systemic pressor effects. The same experiments as in Fig. 2. S.E. values were omitted for simplicity; pressor responses were found to be significant statistically /$p < 0.05$/ for each phase of experiment and for each dose of noradrenaline, except the smallest doses /0.125 µg/kg/.

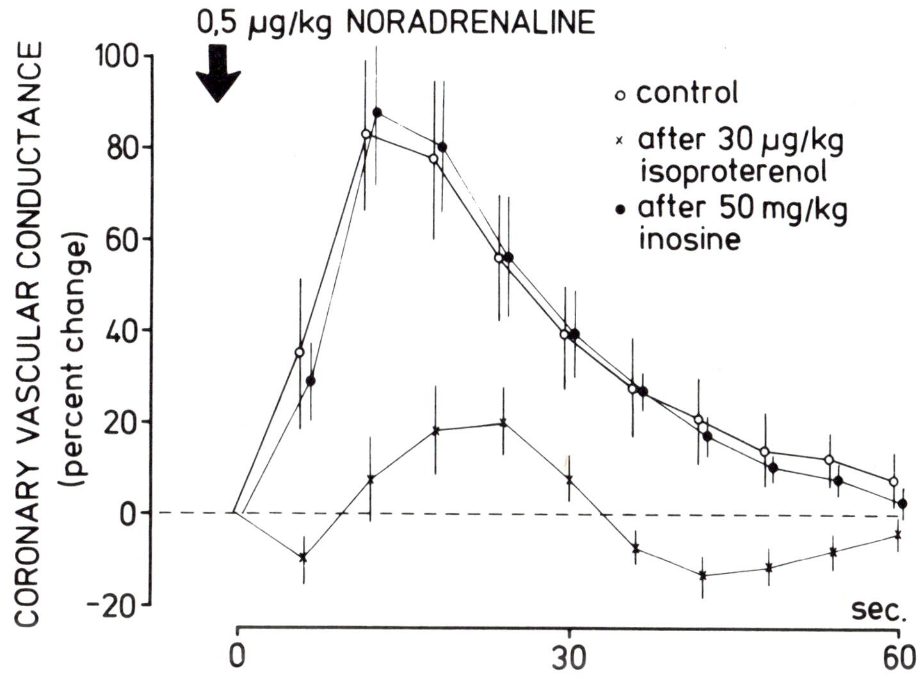

Fig. 4.   Time course of noradrenaline effects induced by
a medium dose. Mean values + S.E.
After treatment with a massive isoproterenol dose
no significant vasodilation was observed except
in the 24th sec of noradrenaline action.
The small coronary vasodilator phase was preceded as well as followed by an equally small vasoconstriction /decrease of calculated coronary vascular conductance/.
n=6

response of isoproterenol can be converted to a vasopressor
effect by previous treatment with various sympathomimetic
amines including isoproterenol and phenylephrine. Since these
agents activate both alpha and beta adrenoceptors, it seems
that beta responses are more easy to desensitize than their
alpha counterparts. Contrary to the above studies, in the
present experiments treatment with isoproterenol did not affect significantly the general circulatory effect of catecholamines exerted on the systemic blood pressure /Fig. 3./.
Accordingly, the desensitizing process appeared to be confined
to some selected portions of the cardiovascular system.
However, isoproterenol doses employed in these experiments
were much smaller than those used by Walz et al. Along these
same lines it could be concluded that a wide variation is present in the propensity for tachyphylaxis among the various adrenoceptors of the circulatory system, and that those localized in the coronary tree are particularly disposed towards
tachyphylaxis.
The inhibitory action on challenging doses of catecholamines
of prolonged exposure to the same agents has led to various
attempts at specify the underlying mechanism for this phenomenon. Although there are several theories, the mechanism is
not clear. This type of desensitization, usually referred to
as tachyphylaxis, seems to be a common, /although not univer-
sal/ characteristic feature of drug-receptor interactions.
Hence, the phenomenon is suggestive of a fairly similar cellular pattern common in a wide range of biologically active
substances.Considering the reversibility of the phenomenon,
tachyphylaxis is likely to depend upon a conformational alteration of receptors. The latter change is probably associated
with an unduly tight agonist-receptor interaction. An increasing number of recent evidences indicate that adrenoceptors
are not merely fixed "patches" at the surface of the cell membrane; in contrast, they are dynamic macromolecular entities
which can be modified by a variety of interventions. Purine
nucleotides seem to be important agents in this respect. It
has recently been demonstrated that purine nucleotides, especially guanosine triphosphate /GTP/ and its analogues profoundly increase the apparent affinity of adrenergic agonists
for catalytic /adenylate cyclase/ activities of beta-type,
without significantly affecting basal catalytic activity
/Williams and Lefkowitz 1978/. The sophisticated nature of the
regulatory nucleotide effect is indicated by the apparent par-
adox of the simultaneous reduction in the agonist affinity for
occupying adrenergic binding sites in the presence of GTP.
Another feature of regulatory action of purine derivates is
exemplified by the surprising finding of former studies, that
an almost complete reversal of cardiac beta-blockade could be
achieved with inosine treatment. Inosine, the first breakdown
product of adenosine which is released in substantial amounts
by the hypoxic myocardium, formerly has been reported to exert
no appreciable cardiovascular effects. However, as early as
1959 Buckley et al. observed that inosine definitely improves
of the contractions of the failing cardiac muscle. This observation was amply confirmed by later studies and extended to the

normal heart. Buckley assumed that improved myocardial contractility was mediated through catecholamine release. The cardiac
effect of inosine is apparently related to that of catecholamines. However, it is difficult to recocile Buckley's assumption with our former /Juhász-Nagy and Aviado, 1977/ and recent
findings, since we have found a practically equal restoration
of the impaired beta-effects elicited either by the exogenously administered adrenergic transmitter or by sympathetic nerve
stimulation. Moreover, recent evidence shows that in the canine
heart the noradrenaline level of the coronary sinus blood is
not affected considerably by inosine administration /Kiss and
Juhász-Nagy, unpublished/. This suggest a mechanism quite distinct from the catecholamine economy of sympathetic nerve
endings, particularly from the regulation of their transmitter
output. More work needs to be done, however, to clear up the
nature of catecholamine-inosine interactions.

Summary

Tachyphylaxic desensitization of coronary beta-adrenoceptors
was studied in open chest dogs narcotized with pentobarbital
sodium. Adrenergic coronary vasodilation was challenged by
supramaximal sympathetic stimulation of the ansa subclavia and
noradrenaline /0.125-2.0 /ug/kg i.v./ administration. Infusion
of isoproterenol /1 /ug/kg/min for 20-30 min i.v./ significantly decreased adrenergic sensitivity of the coronaries characterized by the increase of calculated vascular conductance.
Inosine administration /50 mg/kg i.v./ produced an immediate
reversal of tachyphylaxis. The phenomenon is suggestive of a
possible regulatory role of the nucleoside in adrenoceptor
sensitivity.

References

Butterworth, K. R.: The beta-adrenergic blocking and pressor
    actions of isoprenaline in the cat. Brit. J. Pharmacol.
    21: 378-392, 1963

Buckley, N. M., Tsuboi, K. K., and Zeig, N. J.: Effect of
    nucleosides on acute left ventricular failure in the iso-
    lated dog heart. Circ. Res. 7: 847-857, 1959

Juhász-Nagy, A. and Aviado, D. M.: Inosine as a cardiotonic
    agent that reverses adrenergic beta-blockade. J. Pharmacol.
    exp. Ther. 202: 683-695, 1977

Walz, D. T., and Maengwyn-Davies, G. D.: The mechanism of iso-
    proterenol vasomotor reversal by phenylephrine. J. Pharma-
    col. exp. Ther. 129: 208-213, 1960

Walz, D. T., Koppanyi, T., and Maengwyn-Davies, G. D.: Iso-
    proterenol vasomotor reversal by sympathomimetic amines.
    J. Pharmacol. exp. Ther. 129: 200-207, 1960

Williams, L.T., and Lefkowitz, R. J.: Receptor binding stud-
    ies in adrenergic pharmacology. Raven Press, New York, 1978

<u>Discussion</u>

<u>Rubányi</u>: Irrespective of the mechanism of action, your results
seem to indicate that inosine is a positive inotropic agent.
Am I right in assuming that inosine can be considered as a potentially useful therapeutic drug by which the adrenergic sensitivity can be modulated?

<u>Papp</u>: Being a cardiac surgeon, I hope that the problem I have
studied is not only of theoretical interest but also carries a
clinical significance. It is known that in cardiac surgery,es-
pecially after a cardiopulmonary bypass of considerable duration, some patients fail to respond to inotropic therapy with
catecholamines. This problem continues to occur despite advances of myocardial protection during open-heart surgery. In
fact, some of the described elements of tachyphylaxis may well
be involved in the above unresponsiveness.
Further, the imbalance between myocardial O_2 demand and adequate coronary blood supply to the heart muscle is likely to
ensue under these circumstances, contributing to the deterioration of cardiac performance. It is possible that infusion of
inosine may benefit the depressed myocardium by increasing
coronary vascular adaptation toward normal, and in this manner,
could be helpful in reversing exhaustion of the jeopardized
heart muscle.

<u>Riemersma</u>: Could tachyphylaxis be prevented by inosine admin-
istered <u>before</u> the desensitizing procedure?

<u>Papp</u>: We have not tried that as yet. In our investigations the
exhaustion of beta-vasodilation with isoproterenol was always
established as a first step. Subsequently inosine resensitized
the thwarted response. I welcome your suggestion about reversing
the order of drugs.

COMPARATIVE MORPHOLOGICAL INVESTIGATIONS OF LOCALIZED EXOGENOUS ADENOSINE IN HEART MUSCLE

P. Sótonyi and V. Kékesi

Department of Forensic Medicine and National Institute of Vascular Surgery, Semmelweis University Medical School, Budapest, Hungary

Introduction

Adenosine, an ubiquitous breakdown product of adenine
nucleotide metabolism has been reported to exert various
regulatory functions in the heart such as modulation of
adrenergic neuroeffector transmission /WESTFALL,1977/ and
adjustment of coronary blood flow to augemented myocardial
oxygen needs. The theory concerning the latter function
championed by BERNE since the early sixties /BERNE,1963/
holds that this nucleoside is the key metabolic regulator
of myocardial blood flow not only under hypoxic but under
physiologic conditions of increased cardiac oxygen demand.
Previous pharmacologic studies suggest that adenosine binds
to and acts on specific receptors located superficially on
cellular membranes of myocardial cells and coronary myocytes
/SCHRADER et al.,1977/. In this paper we report the adap -
tation of a new histochemical method described by ROMHÁNYI
et al. which is useful for demonstration of exogenous
adenosine administered in pharmacologic doses /ROMHÁNYI et
al.,1974/, since there is no satisfactory morphological
method or investigation of adenosine binding.

Materials and Methods

The investigations were conducted on mongrel dogs /8-12 kg/
anesthetized with pentobarbital sodium. The animals were

artificially ventilated with room air.After opening the chest
in the fourth left intercostal space a canule was introduced
into the left atrium. Adenosine was administered through this
canule as a bolus injection in a dose of 2.5 - 7.5 /uM dis-
solved in P.S. solution. After adenosine administration the
heart was taken out rapidly and one part put in liquid nitrogen and other part in cryostat for frozen section. The tissues
for polarization optical investigation were unfixed and investigated in cryostat sections /Cryo-Cat Microtome.American.
Opt.Co/. For the polarization optical investigation the
aldehyde bisulfite-toluidine blue /ABT/ method was used
/ROMHÁNYI et al.,1975/.Polarization optical investigation was
made with an Opton polarization microscope equipped with
different compensators. Electron microscopic methods were
based on silver reduction after CSUKA and SUGÁR /1971/. It
was followed by ultrathin frozen sections /Reichert Om U$_2$-FC
150 ultramicroton/ methods and preservation after BERHARD
/1967/.

Results

Adenosine has a strong basophilia but the effect of metachro-
masia and birefringence were strong. The localization appeared
to be in extracellular connection with the outher side of
sarcolemma membrane /Fig. 1a, b / and capillaries /Fig.2 a,b/.
Glycogen granules were rendered strongly basophilic and
sightly metachromatic by the ABT reaction and strongly granu-
led birefringent. The difference between the polarization
optical findings are useful to the differentiation of extracellular adenosine and intracellular glycogen. Electronmicroscopical investigation also revealed an extracellular
localization /Fig.3a,b/. Electron scattering reaction product
was obtained. Only the metabolization of the nucleotids is
fast, which makes evalution of the reaction more difficult.

Discussion

The ABT reaction was introduced into histochemistry by
MALININ/1970/ who found that metachromatic basophilic staining
with this method was characteristic of glycogen.

The molecular mechanism of the ABT reaction and ultrastructural basis of the birefringence induced by the oriented binding
of toluidine blue has been outlined /ROMHÁNYI et al.,1974,
ROMHÁNYI et al., 1975/. A new topooptical reaction was de -
veloped for the polarization optical research of vicinal
OH groups. These method is very sensitive and specific. The
method is based on the peroxidation by periodic acid of the
vicina₋ OH groups or amino alcohol groups, of carbohydrates
to dialdehyde groups, which after addition of sodium bisul -
phite, become negatively charged and able to bind toluidine
blue at pH 2.0. This results in strong basophilia of reacting
compounds as well as a strong toluidine blue induced birefrin-
gence.The basis of the topo-optical staining reactions are
characterized by oriented dye binding on micellar textures
may reveal ultrastructural details in biological membranes.
There is electronmicroscopic as well as polarization optical
evidence to indicate a micellar texture of some macromolecu -
lar elements in biological structures. Adenosine treatment
by periodic acid   oxidizes OH groups which in turn could
bind toluidine blue. The method is useful to investigate biologically active carbohydrate components such as adenosine.
The difference between the polarization optical and electron
microscopical findings are useful to the differentation of
exogen adenosine and endogen glycogen.

Summary

The localization of exogen adenosine was investigated morpho-
logically. The topooptical aldehyde bisulfite-toluidine blue
and electron microscopical silver reaction are useful methods.
The localization showed extracellular connection with sarco-

lemma membrane and capillar spaces in the pericapillar area.

References

Berhard,W.: Ultrathin frosen section. Methods and ultrastructural reservation. J.Cell.Biol. <u>34</u>: 757-771, 1967.

Berne,R.M.: Cardiac nucleotides in hypoxia: possible role in
regulation of coronary blood flow. Am.J.Physiol. <u>204</u>: 317-322,
1963.

Csuka,O. , Sugár,J. : Electron microscopic studies on the
specificity of the PA-silver reaction. Acta Morph.Acad.Sci.Hung
<u>19</u>, 233-240, 1971.

Malinin,G.: Matachromatic staining of sodium bisulfite addition derivatives of glycogen. J.Histochem.Cytochem. <u>18</u>, 834-841,
1971.

Romhányi,Gy., Molnár, L., Németh,Á.: Ultrastructural differences in cell membranes of erythrocytes myeloid and lymphoid
cells as shown by topo-optical reactions. Histochem.<u>39</u>, 261-276,
1974.

Romhányi,Gy., Deák,Gy., Fischer,J.: Aldehyde bisulfite-toluidine blue /ABT/ staining as a topo-optical reaction for demon -
stration of linear order of vicinal OH groups in biological
structures. Histochem. <u>43</u>, 333-348., 1975.

Schrader,J., Nees,S.,Gerlach,E.: Evidence for a cell surface
adenosine receptor on coronary myocytes and atrial muscle.
PflügersArch. <u>369</u>, 251-257, 1977.

Westfall,T.C.: Local regulation of adrenergic neurotransmission
Physiol. Rev., <u>57</u>, 659-728.,1977.

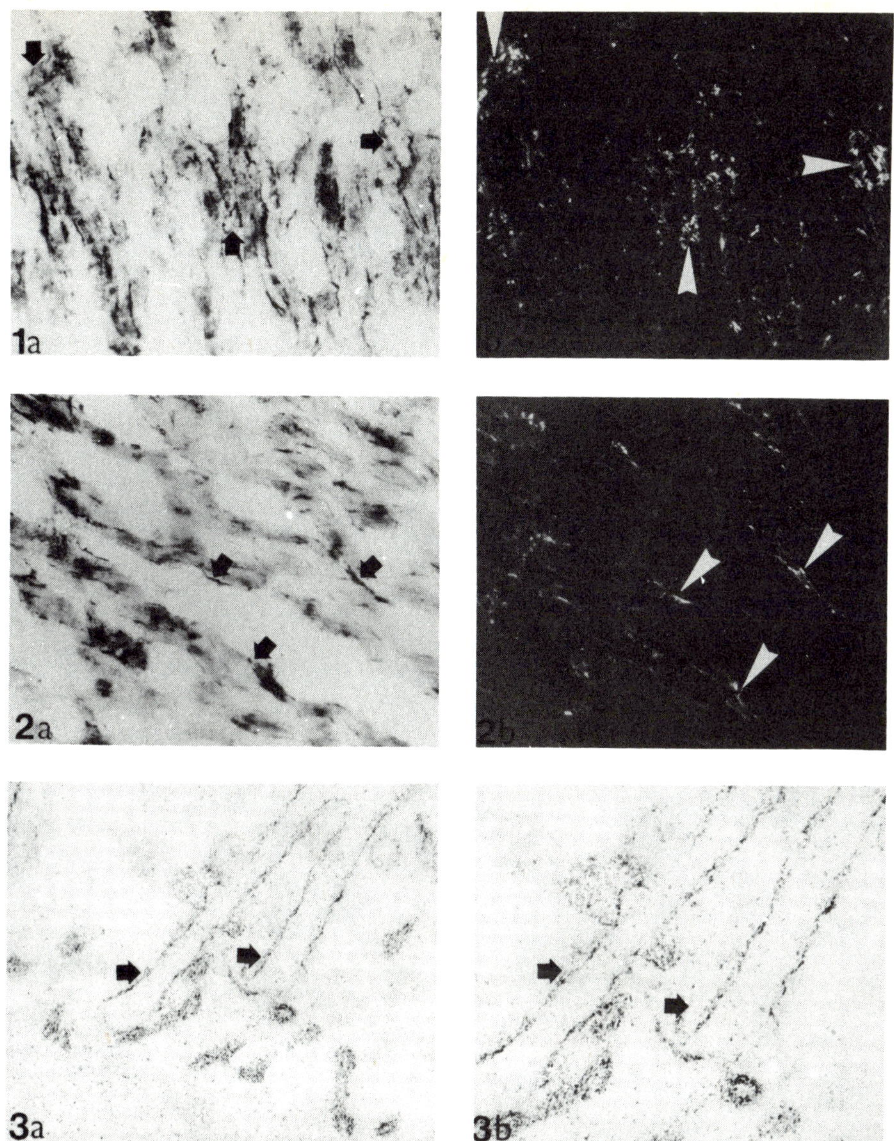

Fig.1 a and b. In the light and polarisation microscope.
The arrows showes the sarcolemmal localization. Magnification 120X

Fig.2 a and b. In the light and polarisation microscope. The arrows
showes capillary localization. /Magnification 120X/

Fig.3 a and b. Electronmicroscopical pictures. The arrows
showes sarcolemmal localization. /Magnification 48000X, 75000X/

117

ADENOSINE SENSITIVITY OF CANINE CORONARIES REDUCED BY CALCIUM-DISPLACEMENT WITH LANTHANUM

Viola Kékesi

National Institute of Vascular Surgery, Semmelweis University Medical School, Budapest, Hungary

There is increasing evidence that adenine compounds (such as adenosine) exert modulatory influences, via a negative feedback regulation, on adrenergic neuroeffector transmission in various tissues (Su, 1977; Westfall, 1977), including heart muscle (Hedqvist and Fredholm 1979; Lokhandwala, 1979). Although the physiologic significance of this modulation is far from clear, it is of great interest that, at the same time, adenosine may also account for metabolic autoregulation in the coronary bed (Rubio and Berne 1975). The intricate sphere of action of adenosine focusses attention on cellular events underlying the coronary vasodilator effect produced by the nucleoside. However, the exact mechanism by which adenosine relaxes vascular smooth muscle is still unknown. In general, contractile responses in each type of muscle are considered to be inseparably related to modified availability of calcium to contractile proteins. The present study was undertaken to examine some effects of calcium on adenosine-induced coronary vasodilation by utilizing the peculiar Ca^{2+}-depleting potency of trivalent La^{3+} ions.

Methods

Mongrel dogs, weighing 15-25 kg, were anaesthetized with pentobarbital sodium (30-35 mg/kg b.w.), ventilated with room air, and instrumented to measure systemic arterial pressure (from a femoral artery) and myocardial blood supply. For the latter purpose the left anterior coronary branch was prepared free and a Statham flow probe

was positioned around the vessel. The probe was connected to a
Godard-Statham SP 2202 electromagnetic flowmeter. Mean flow was
obtained by means of electrical integration. In some cases a Walton-
Brodie strain gauge was sewn to the surface of the left ventricle.
Cardiovascular variables were registered on a direct-writing Hellige
recorder. Drugs were administered into the left atrium through a
catheter introduced into the auricular appendage. Adenosine was either
infused in increasing doses of 8, 15, 30, 60 and 125 μg/kg/min, respectively, to obtain a full dose response relationship, or it was given
as a single bolus (200 μg). $LaCl_3$ was administered in continuous infusions at two different rates: for studying La^{3+} effects due to small
doses, it was infused at a rate of 0.01 mM/min; to obtain results
with larger doses, lanthanum was infused at rates 0.05-0.5 mM/kg
with several temporary interruptions according to the individual sensitivity of the animal. During La^{3+} administrations the adenosine effect
was repeatedly elicited in order to observe the onset and character of
modification in the nucleoside-induced coronary response pattern. Coronary responses were evaluated as changes of calculated coronary
vascular conductance (mean blood flow: mean arterial pressure).
Student's t test was used to compare cardiovascular variables before
and after administration of drugs.

Results
========

Continuous infusion of La^{3+} into the left atrium resulted in decreases of myocardial contractile force, heart rate, pulse pressure,
and arterial blood pressure (Fig. 1.). These effects are similar to
those elicited by Ca-antagonistic agents, such as verapamil, with the
striking exception of the coronary response pattern. In contrast to the
coronary vasodilator action observed after verapamil administration,
La-induced cardiac depression was associated with decreases of coronary blood flow and calculated coronary vascular conductance.
Although this pattern was displayed by each dog I studied, its onset
and rate of development varied considerably from animal to animal.
Consequently, it seemed appropriate to group responses according to

120

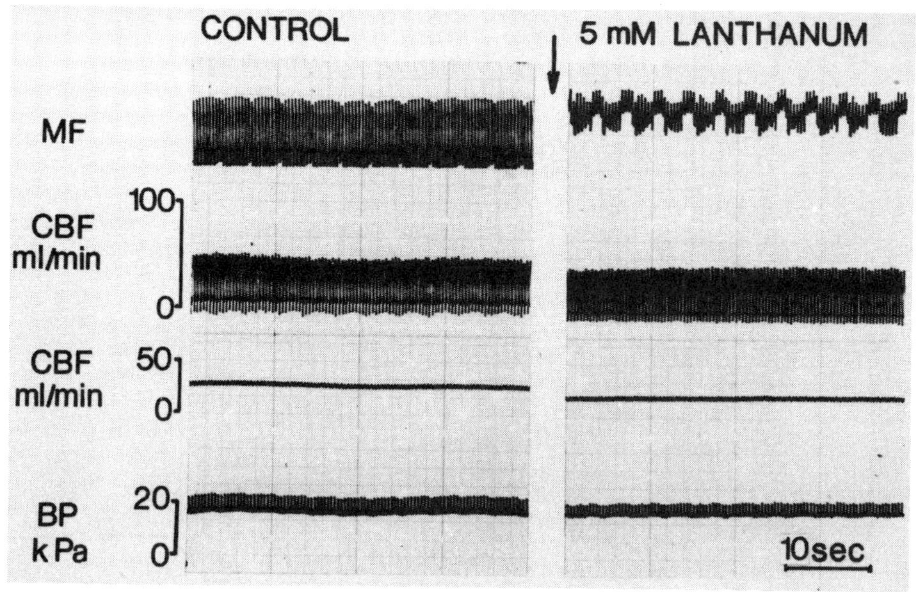

Fig. 1. Effect of a moderate La^{3+} dose on cardiovascular variables. From above downwards: myocardial contractile force /strain gauge/, phasic and mean coronary blood flow, arterial blood pressure (1 kPa = 7.52 mmHg).

fairly broad ranges of cumulative La^{3+} doses. As shown in Fig. 2., when the La^{3+} dose was increased, a parallel trend of vascular conductance decrease could be observed in the coronary circulation. Nevertheless, these coronary vasoconstrictor effects failed to be significant statistically because of their capricious onset and individual time course, i.e. their imperfect temporal coincidence even at the grouping method utilized. At the same time, despite the considerable variability of La^{3+} effect on coronary circulation, the adenosine-induced coronary vasodilation was modified in a characteristic manner. The principal finding was the blockade by La^{3+} of the coronary vasodilator effect. In a smaller range of cumulative doses (up to 1 mM), La^{3+}

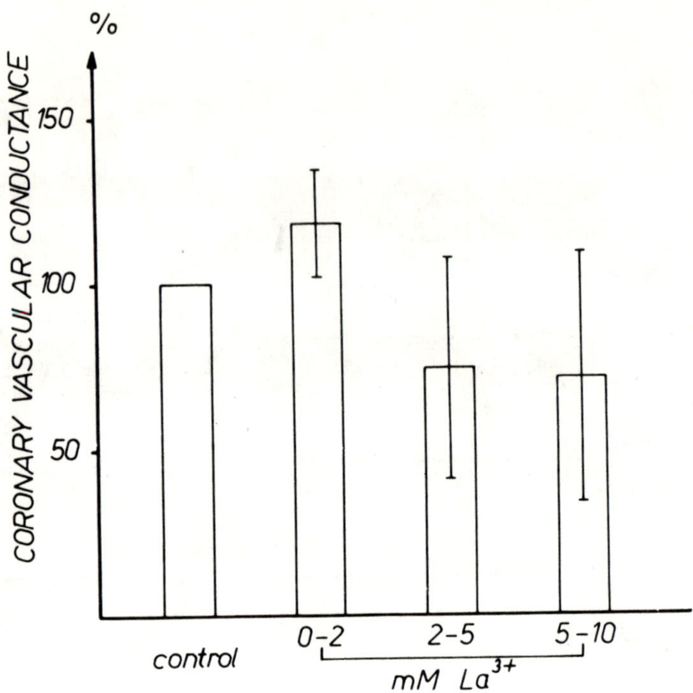

Fig. 2. Effect of cumulative doses of La^{3+} on coronary vessels (n = 7). Vertical bars denote S.E.M.

did not inhibit considerably the adenosine action, although both maximum and steady state c oronary responses to the nucleoside were slightly depressed (Fig. 3.). However, even in this phase I observed conspicuous changes in the time course of the adenosine-induced vasodilation. A typical example is shown in Fig. 4. The records clearly demonstrate a lengthening of the drug-administration to response latency followed by a subsequent delay in restitution of coronary blood flow after the cessation of adenosine administration. The phenomenon is best characterized by the recovery time, i.e. the time in seconds necessary for vasodilator responses (delta vascular conductances) to return to 50 percent of their steady state values (Fig. 5.). Infusions of La^{3+} in increasing doses antagonize the coronary vasodilator action

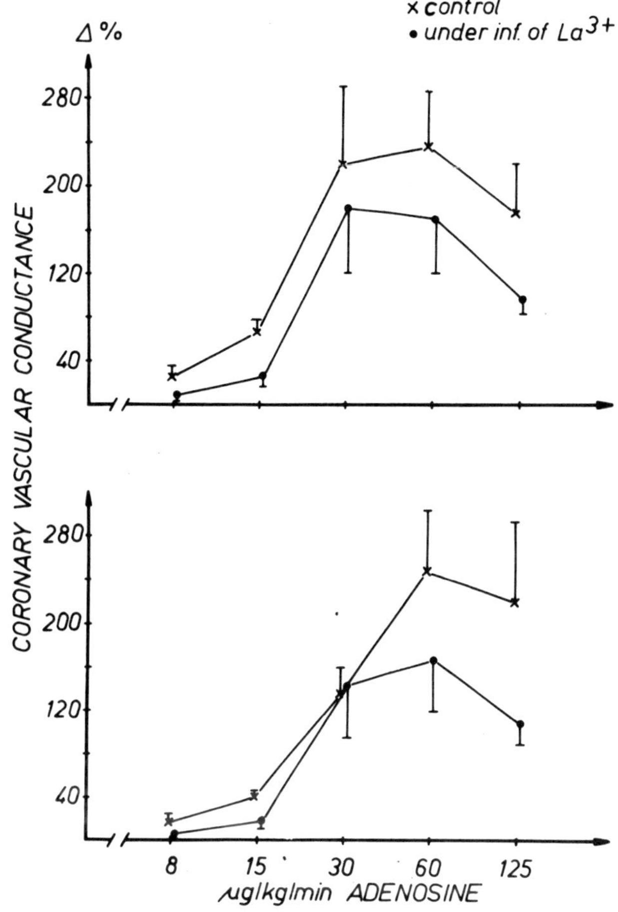

Fig. 3. Effect of small dose of La^{3+} (0.3 - 0.5 mM) on adenosine dose response curves. Maximal (above) and steady state (below) responses during adenosine infusions. Vertical bars denote S.E.M., n = 7.

of adenosine (Fig. 6. and 7.). This effect proved to be dose-dependent and statistically significant. Interestingly enough, the antagonistic effect obtained with the higher doses of La^{3+} was also frequently associated with the lengthening of the adenosine effect.

Discussion

The positively charged trivalent lanthanum ion has the unique potency of displacing calcium from its superficially placed binding sites in the cell membranes. This property of La^{3+} has been utilized ex-

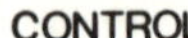

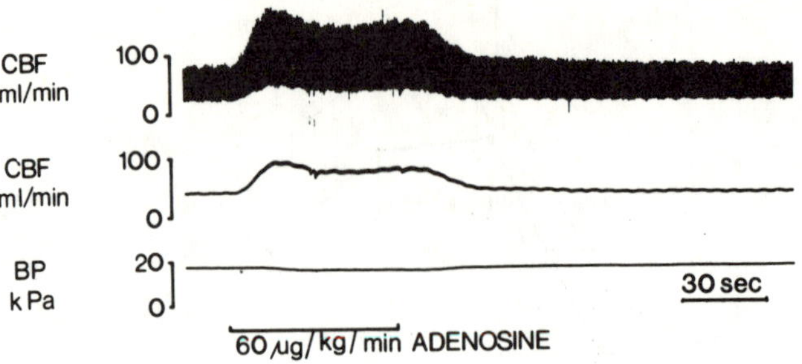

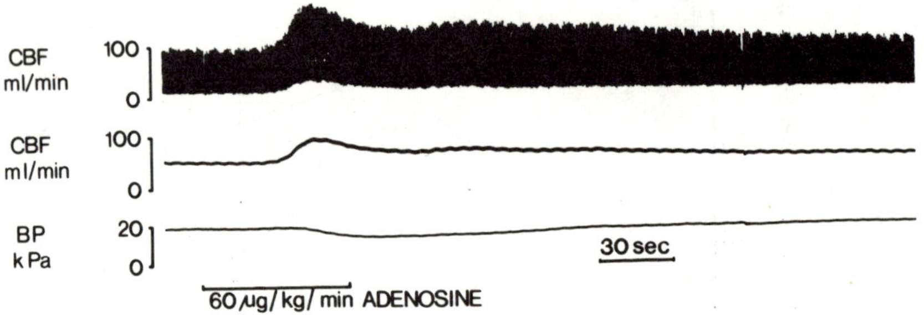

Fig. 4. Prolongation of adenosine effect after La^{3+} administration. From above downwards in both panels: phasic and mean coronary blood flow, mean arterial blood pressure.

tensively for studying calcium distribution in various tissues (for reference see Weiss, 1974). These methods are based on the assumption that, in intact, adequately oxygenated cells, lanthanum does not penetrate intracellularly. At the same time, as it was proposed by Lettwin et al., (1964) lanthanum ions have a higher affinity for calcium binding sites than Ca^{2+} itself. Consequently, La^{3+} not only displaces Ca^{2+} bound to the basement membrane of cells, but exerts a stabilizing action which prevents the entry of Ca^{2+} across the membrane. It is assuemed that in this manner La^{3+} would differentially inhibit responses to various agonists which are dependent upon the extracellular Ca^{2+} pool for activation. Recently it has been shown by van Breemen and Siegel (1980) that unlike aortic (and femoral arterial) smooth muscle,

124

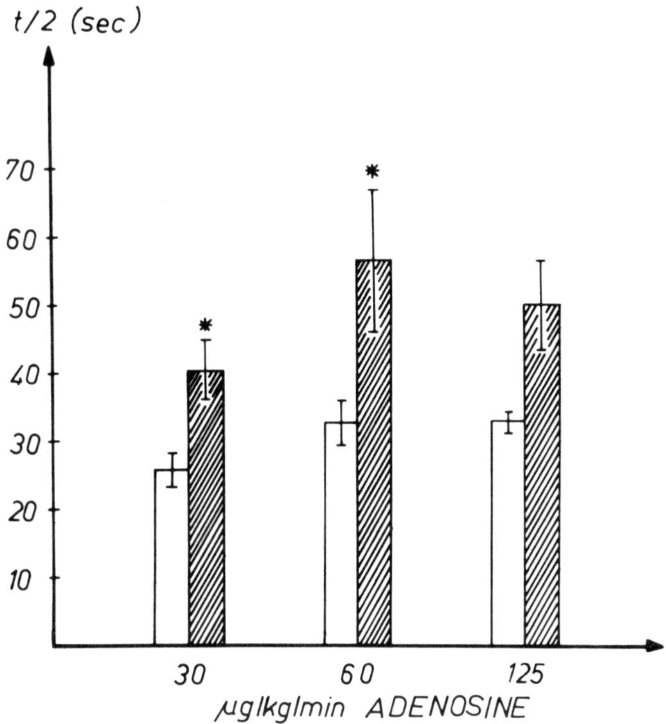

Fig. 5. Prolongation of recovery time of adenosine effect after small doses of La^{3+}. For explanation see text. $n = 7; *p < 0.05$

noradrenaline contraction of coronary arteries is particularly dependent on extracellular calcium: addition of lanthanum in their experiments completely prevented noradrenaline-induced contraction of coronary arteries, but still allowed noradrenaline to produce contraction in other vessels including the femoral artery. In this respect a remarkable parallelism seems to exist between the coronary smooth muscle and the myocardium on one hand, and between the femoral arterial smooth muscle and skeletal muscle on the other, since, like Ca^{2+} antagonistic agents in general, La^{3+} uncouples excitation and contraction in the heart, but fails to do so in the skeletal muscle (Langer et al., 1974).

The most important findings of this study are related to the mo-

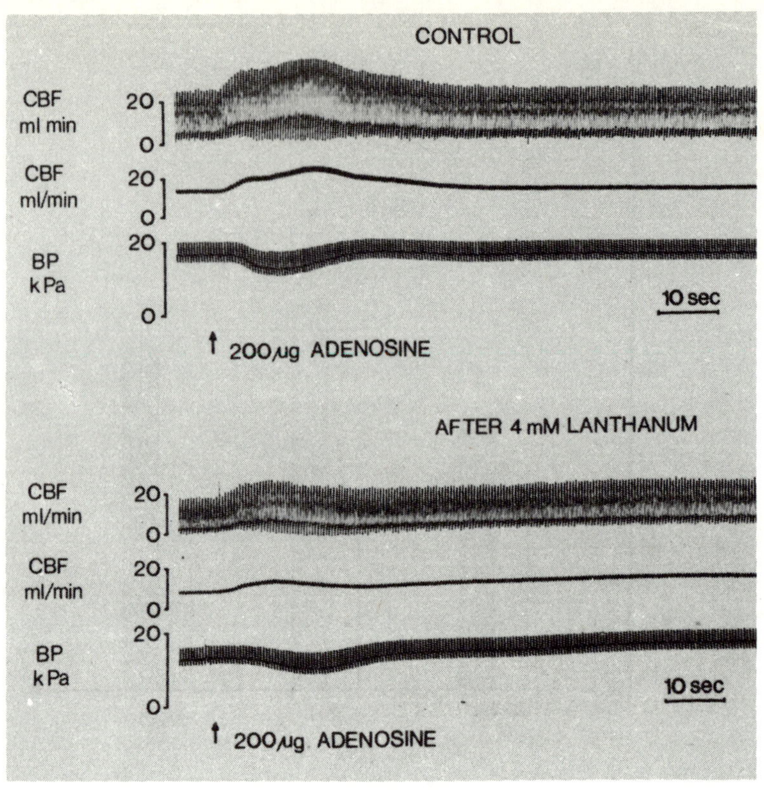

Fig. 6. Inhibition of adenosine effect after 4 mM La^{3+}. Signs as in Fig. 4.

dulation by La^{3+} of adenosine-induced coronary vasodilation. The results obtained could be divided into two categories. The first category includes prolonged adenosine action on coronary blood flow after the administration of La^{3+} in smaller doses. This phenomenon fits well into the generally accepted activation pattern of contractile mechanism in muscle, since adenosine inhibition of the contractile force was shown to be accompained by an inhibition of transmembrane Ca^{2+} influx in atrial muscle (Schrader et al., 1975) and in coronary smooth muscle (Harder et al., 1979). The effect of La^{3+} and that of adenosine may be, therefore, simply additive.

More difficult to interpret the powerful inhibition of adenosine vasodilation after larger doses of La^{3+}. This striking observation, un-

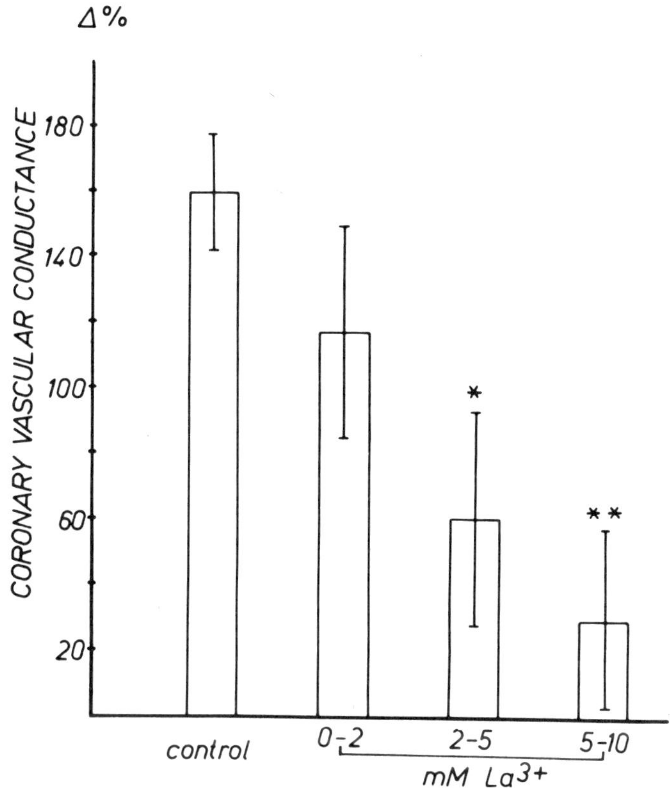

Fig. 7. Dose-dependent blockade by La^{3+} of coronary vasodilation induced by 200 µg adenosine (bolus injections). Vertical bars denote S.E.M. *p $<$ 0.05 * *p $<$ 0.01   n = 6.

expected on the basis of previous current knowledge, suggests a more sophisticated mechanism of action for the "autoregulatory transmitter" adenosine than it has been formerly suspected. At the same time, the present results support the conclusions of recent investigations of this laboratory (Juhász-Nagy, 1980) by verifying the permissive role of extracellular calcium ions not only for activation (vasoconstriction) but also for relaxation (vasodilation) in the coronary bed: it was reported that in the in situ canine heart verapamil inhibits, in a dose-dependent manner, both adenosine-induced coronary vasodilation and meta-

bolic autoregulation simultaneously. The verapamil-induced inhibition
is associated with a vasodilator action of the blocking agent itself,
whereas the La^{3+}-induced inhibition is not. This indicates that the inhibition is adherent to the Ca^{2+} antagonistic action of the blocking
agent rather than to the accidental hemodynamic patterns induced by
verapamil and La^{3+}, respectively. As far as I know, this is the first
time that calcium-dependence of an important vasodilatory mechanism
has been demonstrated, beside the well known dependency upon calcium
of activation vascular phenomena. The explanation for these complex
relationships is not known as yet, but the results suggest that different
cellular functions of vascular smooth muscle may be elicited by, or at
least related to separate pools of extracellular calcium. It is con-
ceivable that adenosine-induced inhibition of transmembrane Ca^{2+} influx leads to accumulation of Ca^{2+} in preferential places on the surface
of vascular myocytes (e. g. in small pockets between the basal membrane and the sarcolemma) thus possibly effecting some kind of membrane stabilization. In that case extracellular Ca^{2+} would be a permissive factor for adenosine action. However, the preliminary character
of the present findings warrant several other, equally possible alter-
native explanations that can only be resolved by further experiments
directed at this question.

Summary

The Ca^{2+}-displacing potency of trivalent lanthanum ions (La^{3+})
was used for studying the Ca-dependency of adenosine-induced coronary
vasodilation in open chest dogs narcotized with pentobarbital sodium.
In smaller cumulative doses (0. 3 - 1 mM, i. left atrium) La^{3+} prolonged the adenosine effect on the coronaries; in larger doses (2 -
10 mM) La^{3+} significantly inhibited the adenosine vasodilation. This
inhibition was associated with cardiac depression and coronary vasoconstriction. It was concluded that the adenosine-induced relaxation of
vascular smooth muscle is a Ca-dependent phenomenon in the coronary
bed.

<u>References</u>

Harder, D. R., Belardinelli, L., Sperelakis, N., Rubio, R. and
Berne, R. M.: Differential effects of adenosine and nitroglycerin
on the action potentials of large and small coronary arteries.
Circ. Res. <u>44</u>: 176-182, 1979.

Hedqvist, P. and Fredholm, B. B.: Inhibitory effect of adenosine on
adrenergic neuroeffector transmission in the rabbit heart. Acta
Physiol. Scand. <u>105</u>: 120-122, 1979.

Juhász-Nagy, A.: Calcium-dependent vasodilation in the coronary bed.
(Abstr.) Proc. XXVIIIth Internat. Physiol. Congr. Budapest,
p. 497, 1980.

Langer, G.A., Frank, J. S. and Tillisch, J. H.: Coupling calcium in
mammalian myocardium: its source and control. In: Reader, R.
(ed.): The Myocardium (Adv. in Cardiol., vol. 12): pp. 162-173,
Karger, Basel, 1974.

Lettvin, J. Y., Pickard, W. F., McCulloch, W. S. and Pitts, W.:
A theory of passive ion flux through axon membranes. Nature <u>202</u>:
1338-1339, 1964.

Lokhandwala, M. F.: Inhibition of sympathetic neurotransmission by
adenosine. Eur. J. Pharmacol. <u>60</u>: 353-357, 1979.

Rubio, R. and Berne, R. M.: Regulation of coronary blood flow.
Progr. Cardiovasc. Dis. <u>18</u>: 105-122, 1975.

Schrader, J., Rubio, R. and Berne, R. M.: Inhibition of slow action
potentials of guinea-pig atria muscle by adenosine: A possible
effect on Ca^{2+} influx. J. Mol. Cell. Cardiol. <u>7</u>: 427-433, 1975.

Su, C.: Adrenergic and noradrenergic vasodilator innervation. In:
Carrier, O. and Shibata, S. (eds.): Factors influencing vascular
reactivity, pp. 156-168, Igaku-Shoin, Tokyo, 1977.

van Breemen, C. and Siegel, B.: The mechanism of alpha-adrenergic
activation of the dog coronary artery. Circ. Res. <u>46</u>: 426-429,
1980.

Weiss, G. B.: Cellular pharmacology of lanthanum. Ann. Rev. Pharmacol. <u>14</u>: 343-354, 1974.

Westfall, T. C.: Local regulation of adrenergic neurotransmission.
Physiol. Rev. <u>57</u>: 659-728, 1977.

<u>Discussion</u>

<u>Leszkovszky</u>: Your experiments appear to show that by substi-
tuting calcium ions in the circulatory system, the total behaviour of the system changes. You have drawn conclusions concerning cellular and subcellular mechanisms from experiments
performed on more or less intact animals, and that seems to me
a rather unorthodox approach to such type of problems. What
grounds, other than lanthanum effect do you have for saying
that extracellular Ca^{2+} is involved in the actions you observed? Have you evidence of similar effects in isolated vessels
or organs? Could you reverse the effect of lanthanum with sur-
plus calcium or otherwise?

<u>Kékesi</u>: The questions you have raised are very important ones.
The involvement of calcium ions was indicated not only by dis-
placement of them by lanthanum, but also by effects of other
agents. In the figure I want to show the infusion of the Ca-
-chelating agent EDTA produced exactly the same pattern as
La^{3+} did in smaller doses. I could not increase the dose of

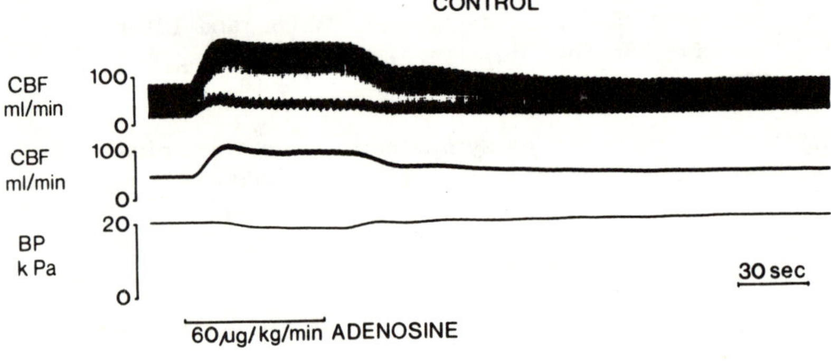

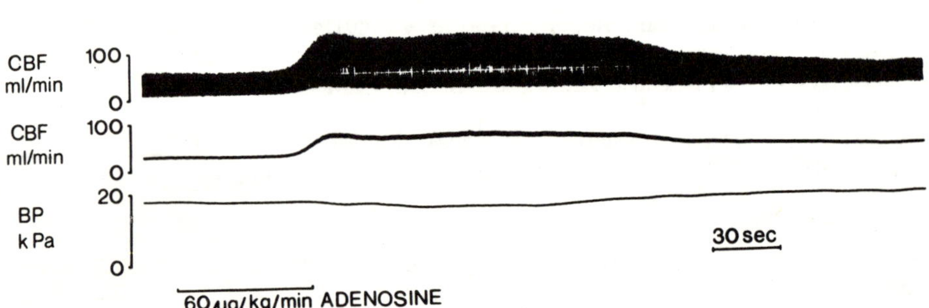

Fig: Effect of EDTA. Signs as in Fig. 4.

EDTA to produce a complete blockade of the adenosine effect
because of the marked hemodynamic effects of the compound,
such as deep hypotension, arrhytmia, etc. However, you can
produce a complete blockade of adenosine-induced coronary vasodilation with the "milder" agent verapamil. In our laboratory
this blockade was found to be reversible after Ca^{2+} administration.

Concerning your second question, I agree with you that
in vitro preparations allow better experimental control and
warrant, in a sense, more valid conclusions about subcellular
events. However, it is very important to establish whether the
physiologic phenomenon that you are studying is not modified
by the procedure of isolation itself. These changes are not
uncommon in the most fundamental coronary reactions. Acetylcholine, e.g. which always dilates the coronary vessels of the
intact heart, contracts coronary vessel wall in vitro. Even
adenosine effect is reported to be absent in isolated coronaries, and sometimes could only be demonstrated after previous
contracture elicited by high concentrations of potassium chloride. In order to keep a proper perspective we tried to remain,
as close as possible, to more physiologic forms of coronary
regulations. Regarding the last problem you raised, i.e. whether the La-effect is reversible with Ca^{2+}, the simplest answer
is that apparently it is not. But, as usual, no simple answer
exists. Much biochemical information is now available about
the kinetics of La^{3+} in biologic systems, and all these show
the unusually strong, practically irreversible character of
binding. In general, my results were compatible with this pattern of binding. Exactly for this reason one is justified to
reckon with cumulative doses in calculations. At the same time,
even at the nadir of cardiac depressions induced by La^{3+}, I
have seen abrupt spontaneous recoveries which indicated an awk-
ward discrepancy between the assumption of the irreversible
La^{3+} binding, and the manifestations of the apparent recovery.
These signs presumably were connected to mobilization of some
"latent" calcium pools, but I must confess that I don't know
the correct explanation as yet.

PHYSIOLOGICAL AND PATHOLOGICAL SIGNIFICANCE OF NICKEL IONS IN THE REGULATION OF CORONARY VASCULAR TONE

Gábor Rubányi, László Ligeti, Ákos Koller, Mária Bakos, Anna Gergely* and Arisztid G. B. Kovách

Experimental Research Department and 2nd Physiological Institute, Semmelweis University Medical School and National Institute of Nutrition, Budapest, Hungary*

INTRODUCTION

Interest in nickel among biochemists, physiologists and clinical scientists has recently increased as a consequence of several fundamental scientific discoveries. It is now well established that Ni is essential for some animals /for Review see Nielsen and Ollerich, 1974, and Schnegg and Kirchgessner, 1976/. Urease has been identified as the first known nickel metalloenzyme /Gordon et al., 1978/.Epidemiological studies have confirmed the long established observation that exposure of nickel refinery workers to certain nickel compounds is associated with increased risk of lung cancer /Doll et al.,1977; Kreyberg, 1978/.The relationship between dietary intake of nickel and exacerbations of nickel dermatitis has been established /Kaaber et al., 1978/. The major role of the kidney in the excretion of nickel /Gitlitz et al., 1975/ and the polycythemia that occurs in rats after intrarenal injection of nickel /Hopfer et al., 1978/ have created interest in the effects of nickel on the kidney.Parenteral nickel prolongs and intensifies the antidiuretic effect of pituitary extracts in rats /Noble et al., 1939/, has an adverse effect on the hypertensive action of epinephrine /Hermann et al., 1954/, inhibits prolactin secretion /Labela et al., 1973/   increases plasma glucose and glucagon levels in the rat /Horak and Sunderman, 1975/ and increases plasma lipid level /Fiedler and Hermann, 1971/.
Nickel can substitute for calcium in certain steps of the excitation-contraction /E-C/ coupling of isolated skeletal muscle /Fischman and Swan, 1967; Frank, 1962; Fuchs et al,1970/ and of the isolated nerve cell /Blaustein and Goldman, 1968; Hafeman, 1969/. A competitive antagonism between Ni and Ca was demonstrated in cardiac tissue /Kohlhardt et al., 1979/ and other investigators suggested that Ni competes with Ca at some membrane sites in the isolated rat heart /Ong and Bailey, 1973; Nayler, 1965/. It has been postulated that Ni can substitute for ·/skeletal muscle, nerve cell/ or compete with Ca /cardiac muscle/ in its binding sites in the plasma membrane Until recently there were no attempts to study the effects of Ni on smooth muscle cells.

The possible significance of trace metals in coronary heart diseases was first proposed by Wester /1965/ who demonstrated a significant disturbance of trace element balance in the infarcted myocardium of human cadavers. The findings that serum Ni level increased significantly in patients with acute myocardial infarction /D'Alonzo and Pell, 1963; McNeely et al. 1971; Nomoto and Sunderman , 1970; Sunderman et al., 1972/ acute stroke /McNeely et al.,1971; Sunderman et al., 1972/, acute burns /McNeely et al., 1971/ and in women with toxemia of pregnancy /Leonov et al., 1971/ suggested that Ni may have some pathological significance in the above diseases.

The pharmacological Ni doses /1 to 10 mM per litre/ used in the earlier experiments exceeded the actual serum Ni level found in patients by a factor of 10^3 to 10^4. In order to gain informations about the possible physiological/pathological actions of Ni it was mandatory to study the effect of much lower Ni concentrations as well. This promted us to analyse the effect of trace amounts of $NiCl_2$ on contractility, metabolism, coronary circulation and ultrastructure of isolated rat hearts /Rubányi et al., 1979, 1980; Kovách et al., 1979, 1980/. It was shown that Ni inhibits cardiac contractility and oxidative metabolism in a dose-dependent manner. However, the most interesting finding was that Ni induced coronary vasoconstriction in a dose as low as 10^{-6} M per litre. In addition a new cytochemical method was found to localize Ni in myocardial and coronary vascular smooth muscle cells /Rubányi et al., 1980a, 1980b/. Trace amounts of Ni were reported to cause structural damages in the myocardium /Rubányi et al., 1980 /.

The present study was designed 1. to analyse further cardiovascular actions of exogenously administered $NiCl_2$ in the isolated perfused rat heart and in the in situ dog heart; 2. to study the possible action mechanism of Ni-induced coronary vasoconstriction; 3. to localize the source/s/ of endogenous Ni release in experimental hemorrhagic shock in the rat and 4. to determine myocardial Ni release under normoxic and ischemic conditions in the dog.

MATERIAL AND METHODS

A. Isolated rat heart

White Wistar rats of either sex weighing 200 to 300 grams were decapitated by a guillotine after intraperitoneal injection of heparin /5 IU per g body weight/. Hearts were rapidly removed and the aortic stump cannulated to allow retrograde coronary perfusion /modified Langendorff technique/ by Krebs-Henseleit bicarbonate buffer solution /KHB/ containing 10 mM glucose and 10 mU/ml insulin. The hearts were perfused by a constant flow peristaltic pump /Watson-Marlow/ via bubble-trap, thermostate /37 ^{O}C/ and filter.

134

A 20 g stainless steel needle was introduced into the left
ventricle through the apex of the heart and connected to a
Sanborn 265 BC pressure transducer. Left ventricular pressure
development /LVPD/ was calculated from the difference of systolic /LVSP/ and diastolic /LVDP/ pressure values. Mean perfusion pressure /PP/ was measured just above the heart via a
Statham transducer. Coronary flow was determined by collecting
all of the effluent fluid in a syringe beneath the heart. All
parameters were recorded on a Harvard Type 490 polygraph.
Total coronary resistance /TCR/ and coronary conductance were
calculated.

B. In situ dog heart

Mongrel dogs of either sex weighing 16 to 33 kg were anesthetized by glucochloralose /100 mg per kg body weight/ with
additional anesthetic given as needed to maintain a constant
level of anesthesia. The animals were immobilized by flaxedyl
/2 mg.kg^{-1}/ and pulmonary ventilation was accomplished by a
positive pressure respirator /Harvard/ with room air en-
riched by 100 % oxygen. Blood gases and pH were monitored
/Radiometer Copenhagen, Type ABL 1/ and they were kept within
acceptable ranges.

A femoral artery and vein were cannulated for continuous
monitoring of mean arterial blood pressure /MABP/ via a
Statham P23HC pressure transducer and for intravenous administration of fluids and drugs. The heart was approached
through a midsternal incision. An electromagnetic flow probe
/Statham Sp2202/ was placed around the ascending aorta to
measure cardiac output /C.O./, around the left anterior descending /LAD/ coronary artery for monitoring coronary blood
flow /CF/ and around the right femoral artery to measure
hind limb /femoral/ blood flow /FF/. Flow rates were measured
by a Statham flow meter.
The flow probes were calibrated in situ by cannulating the artery and pumping the dog's own blood through it at various
known rates by a constant flow peristaltic pump /Harvard/.
Conventional /lead II/ and epicardial ECG were monitored
and spontaneous heart rate was continuously recorded by an
integrator fed by the R-wave signal of ECG. Left ventricular
pressure was measured by a stainless steel needle inserted
into the left ventricle /fixed by atraumatic sutures to the
epicardium/ via Statham P23HC transducer. Dp/dt was continuous
ly recorded by a derivative circuit fed by the ventricular
pressure signal. All of the above parameters were recorded
on a 12-channel Grass Type 7D polygraph.
Total peripheral resistance and vascular conductances
were calculated from the measured hemodynamic and flow
parameters.

Coronary autoperusion

The main left coronary artery was cannulated with a modified
Gregg cannula. The coronary vascular bed was perfused by blood
from the left common carotid artery. The perfusion tubing also
contained an extracorporeal electromagnetic flow probe /Stat-
ham Sp2202/, a side arm for measurement of proximal coronary
artery pressure /i.e. perfusion pressure/ and a site for
intracoronary drug injection by a Harvard pump.

Coronary venous blood sampling

A polyethylene catheter /1 mm, o.d./ was advanced into one
of the two veins running parallel with LAD coronary artery
for continuous venous blood sampling of the autoperfused
myocardial region. Venous blood was analysed for pO_2, pCO_2,
pH, HCO_3^-, Hb and hematocrit /Radiometer Copenhagen, ABL 1/.

Serum Ni level determination

Coronary artery and venous blood samples /4 to 5 ml/ were
immediately centrifugated at 3000 r.p.m. and the serum was
separated from blood cells. Measurements of serum Ni concentration was performed by atomic absorption spectrofoto-
metry /Perkin Elmer 403/ according to the IUPAC recommenda-
tions /Sunderman et al., 1980/.

C. Experimental hemorrhagic shock in the rat

The rats received heparin after pentobarbital anesthesia
/5 mg per 100g body weight/ and both left and right femoral
arteries were cannulated. One of these was used for continuous monitoring of arterial blood pressure and the other
for bleeding of the animal into a polyethylene reservoir until mean arterial pressure reached 35 mm Hg /Rubanyi et al.,
1980/. This low pressure was maintained for 2.5 hours by
regulating the amount of blood given up by the animal. After
2.5 hours the blood was retransfused and 10 minutes later
blood samples and various organs /heart, kidney, liver,
spleen/ were removed for Ni content determination. The
Ni distribution among the same organs and blood was also
determined in control animals, who were anesthetized,
and sham treated for 2.5 hours. Animals in both groups were
fasted for 18 to 24 h prior to Ni determination.

D.Regional myocardial ischemia in dogs

Regional myocardial ischemia was evoked in the in situ dog
heart by mechanical occlusion of the LAD coronary artery.
Arterial and coronary venous blood samples were taken before
/control/ and 1 and 5 min after mechanical occlusion for
serum Ni level determination.

E. Chemicals

The following chemicals and drugs were used in the experiments:
1-norepinephrine /Noradrenalin, Chemical Works of Gedeon Rich-
ter Ltd/; Regitine /CIBA/; Trasicor /CIBA/, Isuprel /Winthrop/;
Verapamil /Verpamil;ORION/; Flaxedil /Specia/ and D-Glucochlo-
ralose /Merck/.

F. Statistical analysis

The mean and standard error of the mean /$\bar{x}$ + SEM/ of grouped
experimental data was calculated. The statistical difference
between means was estimated by the paired and unpaired
Student's t test.

RESULTS AND DISCUSSION

A. Isolated rat heart

1. Dose-response studies

After 30 min of perfusin various doses of $NiCl_2$ were added to
the perfusate in a cumulative manner to reach final concentrations of 0.01-1000 μM per litre. The effect of increasing
$NiCl_2$ concentration on coronary conductance and LVPD is demonstrated in Figure 1. Ni depressed myocardial contractile
force in a dose-dependent manner at high concentrations only
/ above 1 μM/, which is good agreement with previous data obtained on isolated rat heart /Ong and Bailey, 1973/ and myocardial strips /Kohlhardt et al., 1979/.

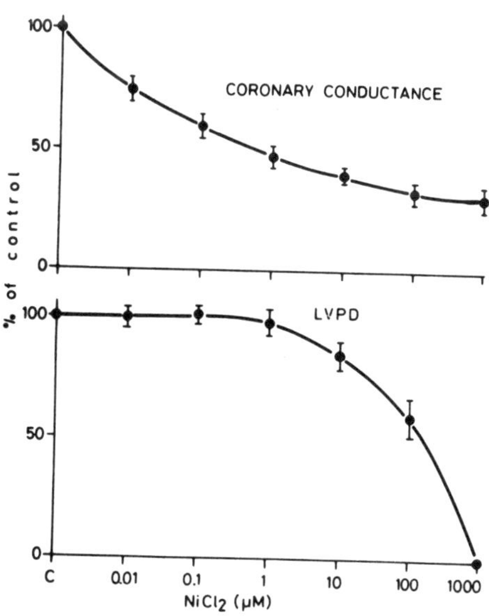

Figure 1. Effect of
$NiCl_2$ on coronary con-
ductance and LVPD of
rat hearts /n=8//$\bar{x}$+SE/

In contrast, coronary conductance was decreased by the lowest
Ni dose /0.01 uM/ already and 1 uM Ni caused a ~50 % reduction
of conductance, when cardiac mechanical activity has not been
altered yet. These results demonstrate that trace amounts of
Ni - comparable to the serum Ni-level found in cardiac patients
- reduce coronary flow considerably, which can not be related
to changes in cardiac contractile activity and thus may be regarded as direct action of this trace metal on coronary vessels. Theoretically this action of Ni may be explained by the
following mechanisms: 1. Ni enhances the influx of Ca into
coronary arterial vascular smooth muscle cells; 2. Ni inhibits
the vasodilatory action of some locally produced metabolite
/e.g. adenosine/ and 3. Ni activates some coronary constrictor
mechanism /e.g. alfa adrenergic receptors/. These possibilities
were experimentally analysed in the isolated rat heart model.

2. Ni-Ca interactions

The addition of $NiCl_2$ to the perfusate abolished LVPD but
caused a 120 % increase of TCR /Figure 2/. Threefold elevation
of perfusate Ca concentration from 1.3 to 3.9 mM restored
myocardial contractile activity and induced a further significant increase of TCR. Thus coronary vascular smooth muscle
reacts to Ni in an opposite direction than cardiac muscle does:
coronary vascular tone was not only enhanced by Ni, but excess Ca potentiated rather than antagonized this effect suggesting a synergism between extracellular Ca and Ni, opposite
to the Ni-Ca antagonism observed in the cardiac muscle. This
finding was further substabtiated by the experimental result
that removal of extracellular Ca totally abolished and prevented the coronary tone increasing action of $NiCl_2$ /Figure 3/.

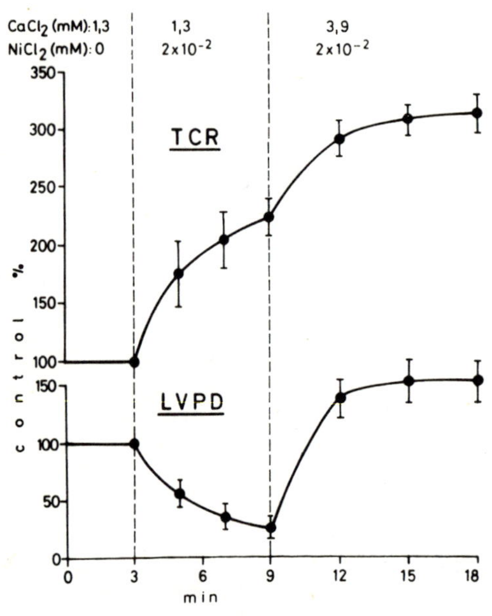

Figure 2. Effect of in-
creased perfusate Ca-
concentration on Ni-in-
duced cardiac and vas-
cular actions. Note
the reversal of LVPD
and further increase of
TCR after threefold e-
levation of Ca-concent-
ration /from 1.3 to 3.9
mM/.

The linear increase of Ni-induced TCR elevation with perfusate
Ca-concentration indicates a firm relationship between extracellular Ca and Ni action on coronary vessels. The experimental finding that the selective Ca-antagonist Verapamil $/10^{-5}$M/
also abolished and prevented Ni induced coronary vasoconstriction /Figure 3/ indicates that Ni enhances the influx /or release from superficial binding sites/ of extracellular Ca
into coronary vascular smooth muscle cells. The exact nature
of this action is totally unknown yet.

Figure 3. The dependen-
ce of Ni induced coro-
nary vasoconstriction
on extracellular Ca
concentration. Note
that Verapamil also in-
hited Ni action in the
presence of 1.3 mM Ca.

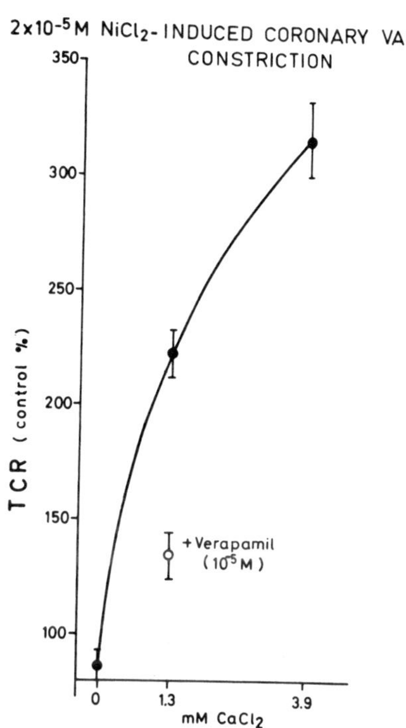

3. Ni-adenosine antagonism

Increasing concentrations of exogenous adenosine /0.1 to 50
/uM per litre/ caused a dose-dependent increase of coronary
conductance in the isolated rat hearts /Figure 4/. 1 /uM Ni
depressed this effect significantly and 10 uM Ni totally abolished it.These results indicate that Ni may inhibit the coronary vasodilating action of locally produced adenosine as well
which may be at least in part be responsible for the coronary
tone increasing action of this trace metal.
The possible link between enhancement of Ca-influx /see above/
and inhibition of adenosine action may be the recent demonstration by Harder et al /1979/ that adenosine, incontrast to Ni,
inhibits Ca-influx in isolated coronary vascular smooth muscle
cells.

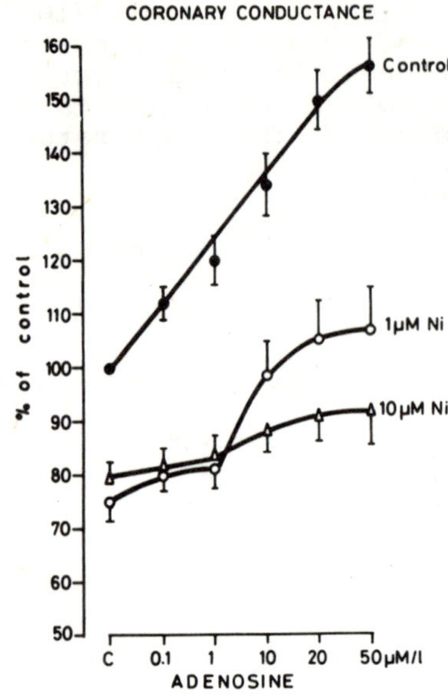

Figure 4. Effect of 1 and 10 μM $NiCl_2$ on coronary vasodilatation of increasing doses of exogenous adenosine in the isolated rat heart.

4. Ni inhibits beta adrenergic coronary vasodilatation

Increasing doses of the beta adrenergic receptor stimulator Isuprel /from 10^{-10} to 10^{-7} g per ml/ caused a moderate but significant increase of coronary conductance in the isolated rat heart in the presence of 10^{-6} g per ml Regitine /Figure 5/. The addition of 1 μM $NiCl_2$ to the perfusate totally abolished coronary vasodilatory action of the drug, at least in the concentration range studied. This finding raises the possibility, that Ni may induce coronary tone elevation by the inhibition of beta adrenergic mechanisms as well.

5. Ni activates alfa adrenergic receptors ?

In the presence of the beta blocker Trasicor /10^{-7} g per ml/ 1-norepinephrine induced a dose dependent coronary vaso-constriction in the concentration range of 10^{-10} to 10^{-7} g per ml /Figure 6/. 10^{-7} g per ml norepinephrine caused a ∼50 % reduction of coronary conductance. After 1 μM Ni induced a similar 50 % reduction of coronary conductance /see Figure 1/ norepinephrine caused only a very slight additional coronary vasoconstriction /15 %/, and 10 μM Ni totally abolished coronary action of the alfa receptor stimulant. The possibilities exist that i. Ni activates /and or occupies/ alfa-adrenergic receptors, or ii. Ni causes a maximal coronary vaso-

140

constriction by a totally different mechanism, and alfa adrenergic stimulation can not increase coronary tone further.
Since the alfa receptor blocker Regitine did not influence
coronary tone increasing action of Ni in the isolated rat
heart /Rubányi; unpublished observation/, the validity of the
latter explanation seems to be possible, but further studies
are needed to elucidate this experimental findig.

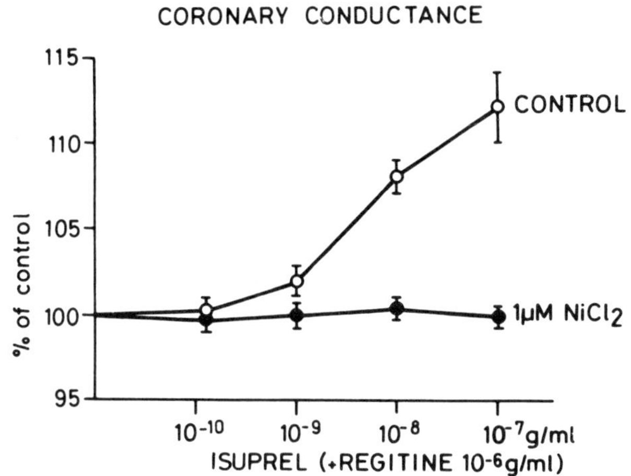

Figure 5. Effect of NiCl$_2$ on beta adrenergic stimulation induced coronary vasodilatation in the presence
of the alfa adrenergic receptor blocker Regitine.

Figure 6.
Effect of NiCl$_2$ on
norepinephrine in-
duced coronary vaso-
constriction in the
presence of the beta
blocker Trasicor.

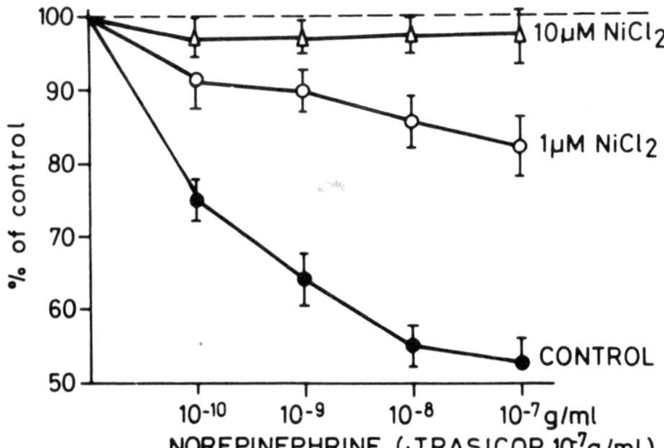

B. In situ dog heart

Increasing doses of NiCl$_2$ /0.02, 0.2 2 and 20 mg per kg body
weight/ were administered intravenously to anesthetized dogs
at 20 min intervals in a cumulative manner and changes of
coronary blood flow, hind limb blood flow, cardiac output,
various cardiac and hemodynamic parameters and of serum Ni
level were simultaneously determined.
The original recording in <u>Figure 7</u> illustrates Ni action on
these parameters. Mean and phasic /late diastolic maximal/
coronary blood flow were significantly reduced by the lowest
Ni dose already, when all other parameters remained constant,
and serum Ni level was also similar to control after 15 min
of bolus injection. The mean values of the changes of these
parameters will be demonstrated and discussed in the subsequent paragraphs.

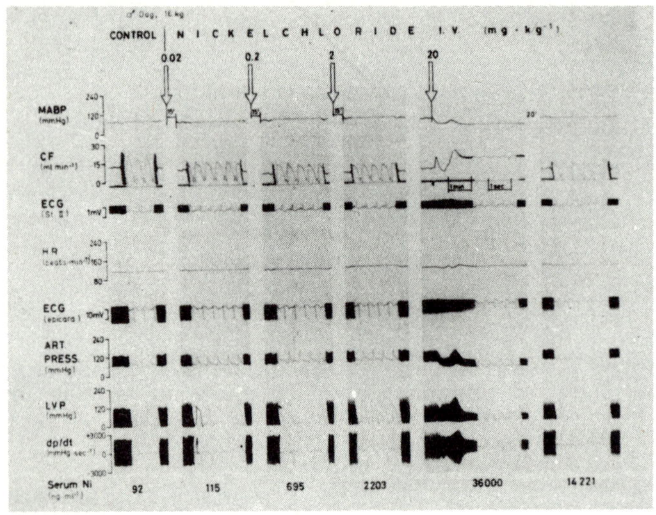

<u>Figure 7.</u> Effect of increasing doses of exogenously
administered NiCl$_2$ on various cardiac and hemodynamic
parameters of an anesthetized dog. Note the significant
decrease of late diastolic maximal coronary blood flow
after the injection of the lowest Ni dose, which did
not induce significant elevation of serum Ni level
/measured 15 min after the bolus injection/.

142

1. Serum Ni level

The lowest Ni dose /0.02 mg.kg^{-1}/ caused a twofold elevation
of serum Ni concentration /from 0.128+0.02 to 0.278+0.03 µg
per ml/ immediately after the injection, but 15 minutes later
serum Ni level returned to control /Figure 8/. At higher injected Ni doses serum Ni level was increased proportionally
and 15 minutes after the injection a considerable decrease
was always observed indicating a rapid elimination of Ni
from the blood.

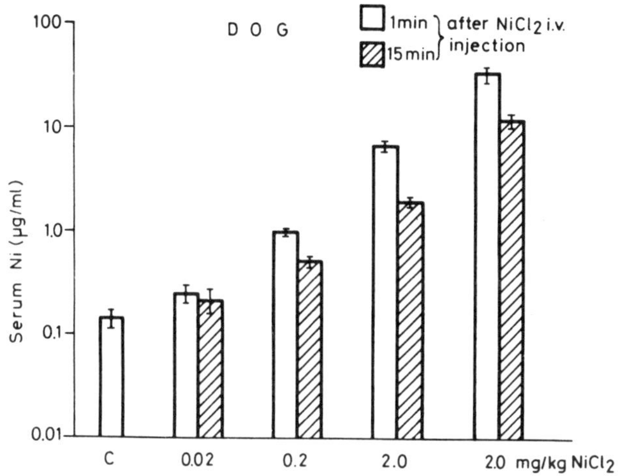

Figure 8.   Serum Ni concentrations of anesthetized
dogs 1 and 15 minutes after the bolus injection /i.v./
of various doses of exogenous NiCl$_2$.

2. Coronary and hind limb blood flow

The lowest NiCl$_2$ dose induced a ∼ 25 % reduction of both
coronary blood flow /CF/ and basal coronary artery conductance
/BC//Figure 9/. Higher Ni doses caused further reduction of
both parameters, thus similar to the results obtained in the
isolated rat heart, trace amounts of Ni caused significant
 decrease of coronary blood flow in the in situ dog heart as
well. Since not only CF but also BC was reduced, the CF decreasing action of Ni may be regarded as the result of local
action on coronary vessels /see also below/.
Similar to CF and BC, femoral blood flow and conductance were also
significantly reduced by increasing doses of exogenous NiCl$_2$
/see Figure 12/.

143

In order to analyse the possible Ni-Ca interaction -
raised by the experimental results on isolated rat hearts
/see Figure 2 and 3/- the effect of the selective Ca-antagonist Verapamil was studied on Ni-induced coronary vasoconstriction in the in situ dog heart as well. <u>Figure 9</u> demonstrates
that Verapamil infusion /0.01 mg.kg^{-1}.min^{-1}/ prior to $NiCl_2$
injection totally abolished the coronary tone   increasing
action of low Ni doses and reversed the action of higher
Ni concentrations /i.e. decreased vascular tone/. These data
together with those obtained in the isolated rat heart clearly
indicate, that exogenous $NiCl_2$ induces coronary vasoconstriction by enhancing Ca-influx into vascular smooth muscle cells
/by a totally unknown mechanism/. The fact that Verapamil not
only prevented but also reversed the coronary action of higher
Ni doses suggests that $NiCl_2$ might induce a decrease of coronary conductance if the dominating vasoconstrictor action is
eliminated.

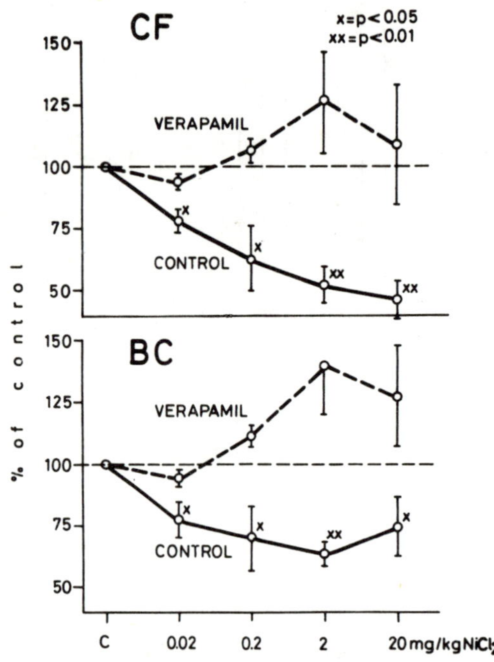

Figure 9. Effect of
increasing doses of Ni
on coronary blood flow
/CF/ and coronary con-
ductance /BC/ of anes-
thetized dogs in the
absence /Control/ and
presence of Verapamil
/0.01 mg.kg^{-1}.min^{-1}/.
Note the absence and
reversal of Ni effect
in the presence of the
selective Ca-antago-
nist.

3. Cardiac performance and hemodynamic parameters

The possibility that the reduction of coronary conductance is
the result of altered extravascular compression due to changes
of cardiac mechanics can be ruled out since neither spontaneous heart rate, nor contractility /dp/dt$_{max}$/ or maximal rate
of ventricular relaxation /dp/dt$_{min}$/ were influenced by low

144

doses of exogenous $NiCl_2$ /0.02 and 0.2 $mg.kg^{-1}$/ /Figure 10/. Higher Ni doses reduced only dp/dt_{min} significantly. Mean arterial blood pressure /MABP/ did not change after the injection of 0.02 or 0.2 $mg.kg^{-1}$ $NiCl_2$, but higher doses caused significant reduction of it /Figure 11/. Total peripheral resistance /TPR/ was not significantly altered in the whole concentration range studied, because the increase of cardiac output compensated the drop of MABP.

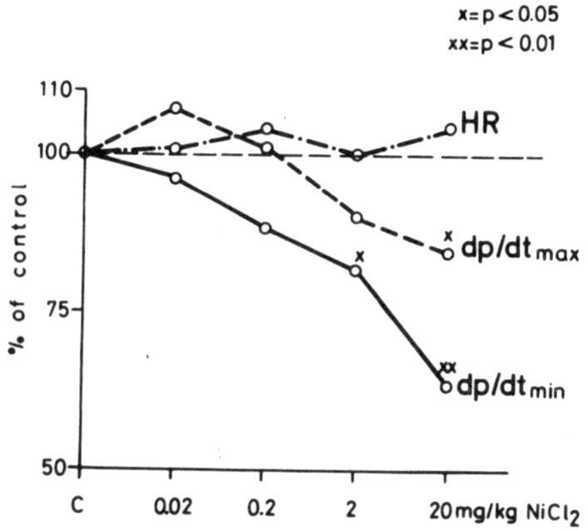

Figure 10. Effect exogenous $NiCl_2$ on cardiac performance /heart rate and contractility/ in anesthetized dogs.

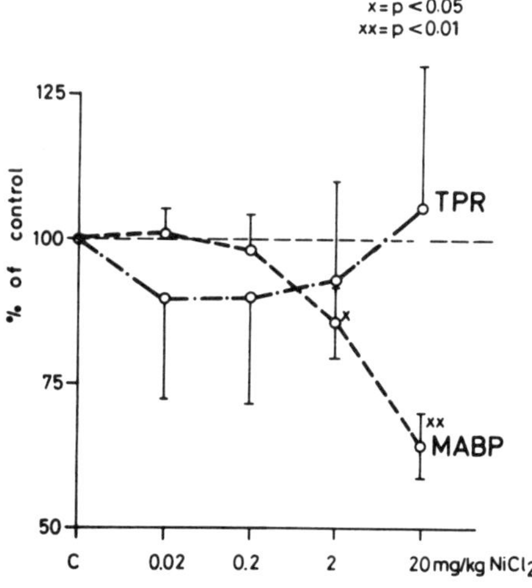

Figure 11. Effect of exogenous $NiCl_2$ on mean arterial blood pressure /MABP/ and total peripheral resistance /TPR/ of anesthetized dogs.

145

These experimental data indicate that in the low /"tracer"/
concentration range exogenous $NiCl_2$ reduces coronary blood
flow without any change in coronary artery perfusion pressure
or cardiac mechanics   suggesting a direct vascular action of
this trace metal.

4. Myocardial reactive hyperemia

Since previous data indicated that Ni acts directly on coronary vascular smooth muscle cells the possibility exists that
Ni may interfere with local regulation of coronary circulation. Reactive hyperemia /RH/ following mechanical occlusion
of coronary arteries was considered to be a suitable model
to yield informatios about local regulation of coronary flow.
/Olsson, 1975/. In order to analyse local coronary actions
of Ni further, the effect of $NiCl_2$ on various parameters of
RH was studied in the anesthetized open chest dog.
Mechanical occlusion of the LAD coronary artery lasted for
10 seconds and it was repeated twice before addition of Ni
/control/ and 1 and 15 minutes after the injection of various
doses of $NiCl_2$. Figure 12   illustrates an original recording.
It is well demonstrated that the lowest Ni dose already decreased the extent of RH, without any change in all other cardiac or hemodynamic parameters. The effect was more pronounced
15 min aftre the injection. Higher Ni doses caused significant depression of RH.

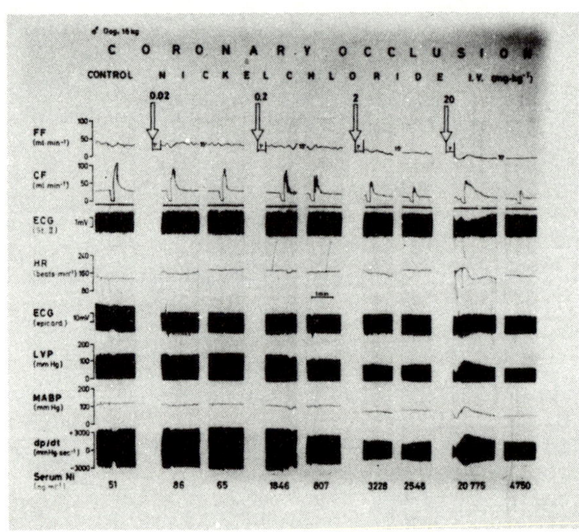

Figure 12.   Effect of exogenous $NiCl_2$ on myocardial
reactive hyperemia following 10 sec mechanical occlusion of LAD coronary artery. Note the significant
depression of the reaction by $NiCl_2$.

146

For further analysis the following parameters were calculated
from the RH response: basal conductance /BC/, maximal conductance /MC/, peak conductance /PC=MC-BC/, reactivity /R=PC/BC/,
the area of flow debt /A_1/ and that of RH /A_2/ and the ratio
of them, the repayment /$R_p=A_2/A_1$/. <u>Figure 13</u> summarizes the
effect of various $NiCl_2$ doses on these different parameters
of myocardial reactive hyperemia. MC and PC did not differ
from control after the injection of 0.02 or 0.2 mg.kg^{-1} $NiCl_2$
but higher Ni doses caused significant reduction of both parameters. In contrast, A_2 and R_p were significantly reduced to
50 % of control by the lowest Ni dose already. These data
clearly indicate that trace amounts of $NiCl_2$ reduce coronary
flow not only under normoxic conditions, but reduce the ability of coronary vessels to dilate under ischemic conditions
as well.

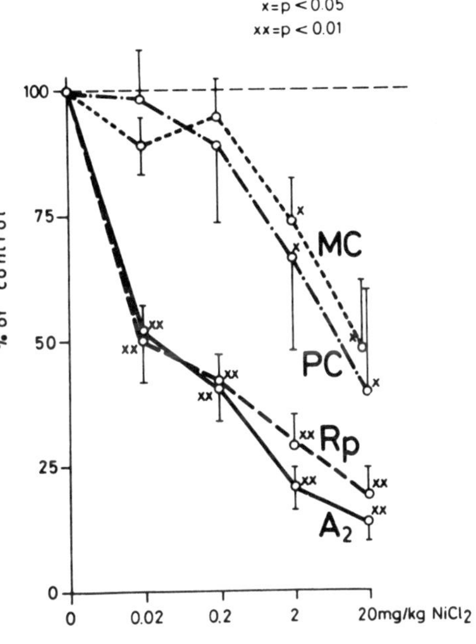

<u>Figure 13</u>. Effect of exo-
genous $NiCl_2$ on various
parameters /see text/ of
myocardial reactive hyperemia in the anesthetized
dog.

The fact that trace amounts of exogenous $NiCl_2$ reduced A_2 and R_p significantly / the two parameters of myocardial RH which correlate best with tissue metabolite /i.e. adenosine/ accumulation during occlusion /Olsson, 1975// indicate that Ni action on RH /and most probably on coronary vessels/ may be explained by the tissue metabolite hypothesis of RH /Olsson, 1975/. On the basis of this hypothesis the possible causes of Ni action are as follows: 1. diminished rate or amount of adenosine production, 2. increased rate of metabolite elimination, and 3. reduced reactivity of coronary vessels. The findings that neither heart rate nor left ventricular contractile performance were altered by trace amounts of Ni indicate that reduced production of adenosine due to depressed mechanical activity or metabolic demands can be excluded with great probability. The time course of tissue metabolite elimination corresponds to the rate of coronary flow prior to occlusion /Olsson et al., 1978/. Since CF was reduced by Ni prior to mechanical occlusion, an increased rate of adenosine washout from the myocardium can not be the cause of Ni action. The third possibility, that Ni reduces CF by antagonizing adenosine action on the coronary vessels, involves the following possible mechanisms: 1. interaction with adenosine receptors, 2. direct vascular smooth muscle activation which antagonizes the action of adenosine. The assumption /based on experimental data obtained in the isolated rat heart/ that Ni enhances Ca-influx into coronary vascular smooth muscle cells and the finding that adenosine inhibits Ca-influx /Harder et al.,1979/ argue for the validity of the latter possible action mechanism. The demonstration that Ni inhibits coronary vasodilatation induced by exogenous adenosine in the isolated rat heart /Figure 4./ underlies this assumption.

C. Endogenous Ni-release from the ischemic myocardium

1. Hemorrhagic shock

During prolonged, severe hemorrhagic shock coronary blood flow becomes inadequate and functional as well as structural myocardial damages develop /Rubányi et al., 1980/, which were reported to be mainly of hypoxic/ischemic origin /Rubányi et al., 1980/. Thus experimental hemorrhagic shock in the rat proved to be a good animal model for studying endogenous Ni redistribution. The change of Ni content in various organs following 2.5 hours of hemorrhagic hypotension /35 mm Hg/ of the rat is demonstrated in Figure 14. Control animals /fasted for 18 to 24 hours similar to that of shocked animals/ exhibited a very high myocardial and kidney Ni content, while that of the serum, liver and spleen was much lower / each measurement was performed on 4 to 8 organs "pooled" from various animals treated similarly/. Serum Ni level was significantly elevated during hemorrhagic shock /from $0.114+0.012$ to $0.294+0.02$ μg per ml; $p < 0.001$/. Tissue Ni content measurements revealed that the main sources of the released Ni were

the heart and the liver, the Ni content of which was reduced
to about 30 % of the control. Ni content of the kidney was
slightly increased, but it was not statistically significant.
The spleen exhibited no change in Ni content.

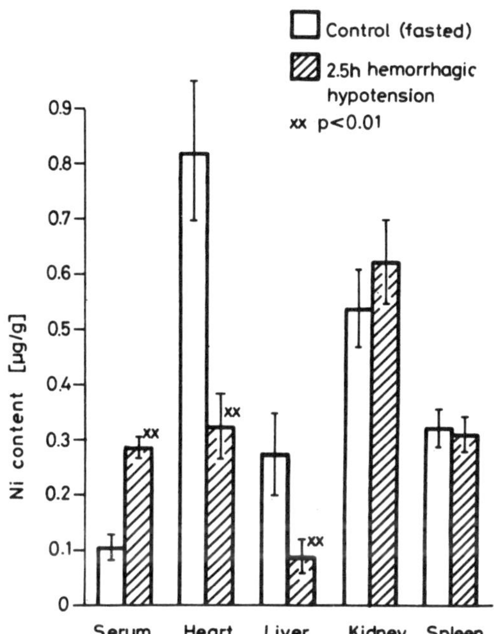

Figure 14. Endogenous Ni redistribution in various organs of the rat /measured by atomic absorption spectrophotometry/ during 2.5 h hemorrhagic hypotension.

2. Regional myocardial ischemia in the dog heart

The measurement of Ni content of the coronary artery and venous blood revealed that under control /normoxic/ conditions
Ni content was always significantly higher in the coronary
vein /Figure 15/ indicating a continuous Ni-release from the
normoxic myocardium /negative AV-Ni difference/. Mechanical
occlusion of the coronary artery for 1 min resulted in a
slight elevation of arterial Ni content but a more pronounced
increase of venous Ni level /viz. significantly increased
Ni-release from the ischemic myocardium/. After 5 min ischemia arterial Ni level increased significantly, but venous Ni
content was reduced, resulting in a positive AV-Ni difference
/uptake of Ni by the myocardium/.

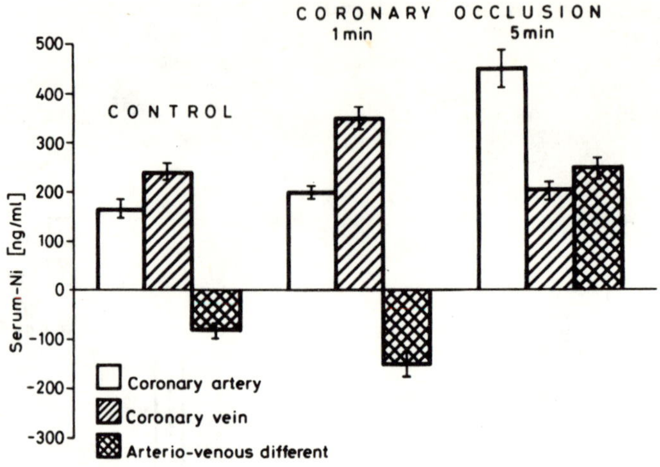

<u>Figure 15.</u>   Coronary arterial and venous Ni level as well as AV-Ni difference in the normoxic /control/ dog heart and after 1 and 5 min mechanical occlusion of the coronary artery /myocardial ischemia/.

CONCLUSIONS AND HYPOTHESES

1.Physiological importance of Ni

The experimental finding that Ni is continuously released from the normoxic myocardium /Figure 15/ raises the possible physiological importance of endogenous Ni. It is suggested that the continuous. /"tonic"/ coronary dilating action of continuously produced adenosine under normoxic conditions / Olsson,1970/ is opposed by the coronary tone increasing effect of endogenously released Ni /<u>negative feed back</u>/. Until now there was no substance known which may regulate /or antagonize/ the coronary vascular tone decreasing action of adenosine. The exact nature of this hypothetical phenomenon needs further investigations in the future.

2. Pathological significance of Ni

During ischemia the heart relies on anaerobic metabolism and tissue hypoxia induces increase of adenosine production and consequently this metabolite accumulates in the myocardium /Berne, 1964/. After release from the cell this metabolite exerts a very intensive local stimulus for coronary vasodilatation. This local vasodilating stimulus is opposed in certain cases /shock, infarction, etc.,/ by the coronary tone increasing action of circulating catecholamines and increased sympa-

150

thetic drive /adrenergic control/, by circulating endotoxins
and by tissue edema /Figure 16/.

The present experimental data strongly indicate that endogenous Ni release may be also a very potent coronary tone increasing mechanism under ischemic conditions. Although nothing
is known to date about the nature of Ni release from the myocardial cells, it is hypothetized that cellular Ni is released
from binding sites and after efflux from the cell reaches coronary arterioles where it exerts   coronary vascular smooth
muscle contraction or reduces the ability of the arterioles
to dilate maximally under hypoxic/ischemic conditions.
As far as the action mechanism of Ni is concerned the present
experimental data indicate the following possible mechanisms:
1. enhancement of Ca-influx into vascular smooth muscle cells,
2. inhibition of coronary vasodilatation induced by adenosine,
3. inhibition of coronary vasodilatation induced by beta-adrenergic receptor stimulation,
4. stimulation of alfa-adrenergic receptor mechanisms/?/.
Excess Ni released from the myocardium produces an elevation
of serum Ni level in combination with Ni released from the
liver /Figure 16/. Ni released in the vicinity of coronary arterioles reduces nutritive coronary blood flow, which leads to
further myocardial damages /positive feed back/.This positive
feed back action of endogenous Ni release is thought to be the
most important pathological action of this trace metal in certain cardiovascular diseases. Thus endogenous Ni release from
the hypoxic/ischemic myocardium, unless prevented or treated,
may lead to cardiac failure.

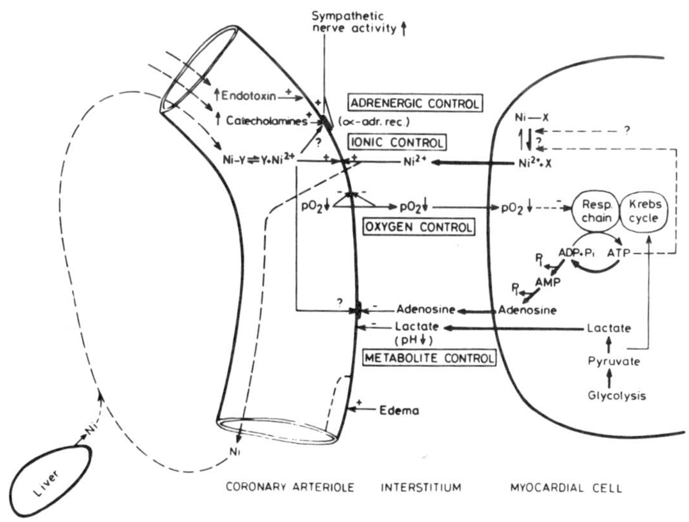

Figure 16. Hypothetical model for the control of coronary
vascular tone in myocardial ischemia /description see text/

SUMMARY

1. Trace amounts /0.01-1.0 μM per litre/ of exogenous $NiCl_2$ reduce coronary flow and coronary conductance in the iso-lated rat heart and in situ dog heart by a local action on coronary vessels.

2. Coronary vascular tone increasing effect of Ni is dependent on extracellular Ca-concentration. Since the specific Ca-antagonist Verapamil prevented and abolished Ni action in both preparations the major action mechanism of Ni was suggested to be the enhancement of Ca-influx into coronary vascular smooth muscle cells.

3. Experimental data provided evidences for a possible Ni-adenosine antagonism in the regulation of coronary vascular tone.

4. Studying the possible interactions between Ni and adrener-gic receptor mechanisms revealed that Ni may increase coro-nary vascular tone by inhibiting beta-adrenergic receptor stimulation mediated coronary vasodilatation and/or by ac-tivating or mimicing alfa adrenergic mechanisms in the coro nary vessels.

5. The finding that Ni is continuously released from the normoxic myocardium raised the possibility that Ni may play important role in the physiological local regulation of coronary vascular tone.

6. Myocardial Ni release was significantly increased during myocardial ischemia induced by hemorrhagic shock in the rat or by mechanical occlusion of the coronary artery in the dog. This finding suggests the possible pathological significance of this trace metal in cardiovascular disea-ses, since released Ni reduces nutritive coronary blood flow which results in further myocardial damages, etc. /positive feed back loop/.

REFERENCES

Berne,R.M. - Physiol.Rev. 44:1, 1964
Blaustein,M.P., Goldman,D.E. - J.Gen.Physiol.51:279,1968
D'Alonzo,C.A., Pell,S. - Arch.Environ.Health 6:381, 1963
Doll,R., Mathews,J.D.,Morgan,L.G. - Brit.J.Ind.Med. 34:102,1977
Fiedler,H.,Hermann,I. - Folia Hematol. 96:224, 1971
Fischman,D.A., Swan,R.C. - J.Gen.Physiol. 50:1709, 1967
Frank,G.B. - J.Physiol /London/ 163:154, 1962
Fuchs,F., Reddy,Y., Briggs,F.N. - Biochim.Biophys.Acta 221:407, 1970

Gitlitz,P.H., Sunderman,F.W.Jr., Goldblatt,P.J. - Toxicol.Appl.
     Pharmacol. 34:430, 1975
Gordon,W.R., Schwemmer-S.S., Hillman,W.S. - Planta 140:265,1978
Hafemann,D.R. - Comp.Biochim.Physiol. 29:1149,1969
Harder,D.R.,Belardinelli,L.,Sperelakis,N.,Rubio,R.,Berne,R.M.-
     Circ.Res. 44:176,1979
Hermann,H.,Chatonnet,J.,Vial,J. - Arch.Int.Pharmacodyn. 98:129,
                                                        1954
Hopfer,S.M., Sunderman,F.W.Jr.,Fredrickson,T.N.,Morse,E.E. -
     Ann.Clin.Lab.Sci. 8:396, 1978
Horak,E., Sunderman,F.W.Jr. - Toxicol.Appl.Pharmacol. 33:388,
                                                       1975
Kaaber,K.,Veien,N.K.,Tjell,J.C. - Brit.J.Dermatol. 98:197,1978
Kohlhardt,M. - J.Mol.Cell.Cardiol. 11:1127, 1979
Kovach,A.G.B., Rubanyi,G., Ligeti,L., Koller,Á.- Fed.Proc.
     39:1215, 1980
Kovách,A.G.B., Rubányi,G. - Physiologist 22:72, 1979
Kreyberg,L. - Brit.J.Ind.Med. 35:109, 1978
Labela,F.S. - Nature 245:330, 1972
Leonov,V.A., Gurskaya,I.K. - Dokl.Akad.Nauk.Beloruss.SSR, 15:
     656, 1971
McNeely,M.D.,Sunderman,F.W.Jr.,Nechay,M.W.,Levine,H. - Clin.
     Chem. 17:1123, 1971
Nielsen,F.H., Ollerich,D.A. - Fed.Proc. 33:1767, 1974
Noble, R.L.,Rindreknecht,H., Williams, P.C. - J.Physiol./London/
     96:293, 1939
Nomoto,S.,Sunderman,F.W.Jr. - Biochemistry 10:1647, 1971
Olsson,R.A. - Circ.Res. 26:301, 1970
Olsson,R.A. - Circ.Res. 37:263, 1975
Olsson,R.A.,Snow,J.A.,Gentry,M.K. - Circ.Res. 42:358,1978
Ong,S.D., Bailey,L.E. - Am.J.Physiol. 224:1092, 1973
Rubányi,G.,Pintér,C., Kovách,A.G.B. - Kisérl.Orvostud. 31:38,
                                                        1979
Rubanyi,G., Koltay,E.,Nagy-Dóra,T.,Balogh,I.,Kovách,A.G.B.,
     Somogyi,E. - Circ.Shock 7:59, 1980
Rubanyi,G.,Balogh,I.,Somogyi,E.,Kovách,A.G.B.,Sótonyi,P. -
     J.Mol.Cell.Cardiol. 12:609, 1980
Rubányi,G.,Kovach,A.G.B. - Acta Physiol.Acad.Sci.hung.-in press
Sunderman,F.W.Jr.,Decsy,M.I.,McNeely,M.D. - Ann.N.Y.Acad.Sci.
     199:300, 1972
Sunderman,F.W.Jr. - Pure Appl.Chem. 52:527, 1980
Schnegg,A., Kirchgessner,M. - J.Vitamin Nutr.Res. 46:96, 1976
Wester,P.O. - AE-188/UDC 616.12:543.53/ Stockholm, 1965

DISCUSSION

Szentmiklósi: I congratulate to your interesting findings especially to the demonstration of antagonism between Ni^{2+} and adenosine as well as norepinephrine. Is there any ligand formation between Ni ions and these substances.

Rubányi: It is well known that Ni readily forms complexes with various substances, but there are no data available at present about possible ligand formation with adenosine or catecholamines.

Riemersma: Is it possible that Ni^{2+} abolishes norepinephrine action simply because it oxidizes the catecholamine in the Krebs solution?

Rubányi: This is another possibility which needs further investigation, since there are no data available in this respect. It is also possible, however, that due to its complex formation ability or oxidizing /etc./ properties, Ni interferes with certain membrane constituents /"receptors"/ which may cause the observed changes in coronary vascular tone and coronary reactivity.

Kunos: Theoretically it is also possible that Ni^{2+} releases calcium from a cellular pool which is essential in the mechanism of alpha adrenergic stimulation.

Rubányi: The dependence of Ni action on extracellular calcium-concentration suggests that coronary vascular action of this trace element is closely related to Ca influx and/or mobilization in the vascular smooth muscle cells. The demonstration of close relationship between alpha adrenergic stimulation and Ca^{2+} validates the assumption raised by dr Kunos. However, van Breemen et al. /1980/ reported that norepinephrine induces contraction in the isolated canine coronary artery /in contrast to the aorta/ by enhancing the influx of extracellular Ca^{2+}. There is no intracellular Ca-release during alpha adrenergic stimulation in the coronary artery.

Kunos: Is the effect of Ni specific, or do other trace metals exert a similar action?

Rubányi: Similar ti Ni, Co ions also induce significant coronary vasoconstriction in the isolated rat heart in 0.1/uM/1 concentration already. There were also reports about coronary vasoconstriction induced by vanadium /V/ /Schwartz et al.,1980/. The systematic analysis of cardiovascular /and especially coronary/ action and interaction of various essential trace elements needs intensive work in the future.

PHYSIOLOGICAL AND PATHOLOGICAL EFFECTS OF BETA MODULATOR RELEASE

M. Szentiványi and G. P. Leszkovszky
Department of Pharmacology, Chemical and Pharmaceutical Works CHINOIN, Budapest, Hungary

In previous studies it could be demonstrated that by increasing the metabolic level of an organ its alpha receptors can be transformed into beta form /Szentiványi et al. 1970; Szentiványi and Kunos 1969/. This transformation takes place by a modulator substance. Accordingly beta receptors equal alpha receptors+modulator substance. Heart being an organ of high metabolic level, constantly synthesizes this substance thus producing beta receptors for itself. Metabolic dilation after catecholamines has proved to be a consequence of beta receptor stimulation./Szentiványi et al. 1970; Szentiványi and Kunos 1969/. It is obvious that this modulator substance synthesized in myocardium is responsible eventually for adrenergic metabolic dilation. If this substance is transferred from myocardium to the coronaries a virtual "autometabolic" dilation of these latters could manifest. In this case coronaries would behave as having beta receptors for their own, nevertheless they possess modulator substance only from the myocardium. If a release and eventually a depletion of this modulator substance can be effectuated either from the myocardium or the coronaries, this problem is easy to solve.

Following this line it could be of interest whether in general metabolic disorders an incompletness of the adrenergic metabolic dilation, i.e. alpha-beta receptor transformation takes place. In the second part of this paper the problem of diabetic angiopathy will be dealt with shortly.

Materials and methods.

<u>Dogs' hind limb preparation</u>. 51 mongrel dogs under urethan-chloralose anesthesia were used. One of the femoral arteries was perfused from the contralateral femoral artery. Flow was recorded by means of an extracorporal electromagnetic flow probe operated by a Statham flowmeter type Multiflow M4000. Sytemic blood pressure /BP/, perfusion pressure were also recorded.

<u>Experiments on heart/coronaries</u>. The flow of the r. circumflexus of the left coronary was recorded by an electromagnetic flowmeter together with left ventricular pressure, enddiastolic pressure, dp/dt, heart rate and systemic BP. The vasomotor changes of the coronaries, uninfluenced by extravascular factors, were determined by enddiastolic resistance.

<u>Diabetic angiopathy</u>. On aortic strips of control and diabetic rats /25 mg/kg-75 mg/kg Streptozotocin single dose/cumulative NA dose-response curves were made. The influence on them by propranolol and a specific blocking substance /NP51/ was studied. This latter acted only on "false diabetic" beta receptors produced in diabetes by a false modulator substance.

Control, spontaneous diabetic and Streptozotocin treated rats were administered NP51 / 5 mg/kg/die / for 2-3 months. After killing the animals, histological sections were made of heart, coronaries, aortae and of mesenteric vessels, as well as of the kidneys. The developed micro- and macroangiopathy were compared with values of the controls. As for microangiopathy vessel-diameters were counted within several ranges and were expressed in %. It was investigated whether in classes of higher wall thickness the number of vessels increased in diabetes and this increase could be prevented by specific drugs.

Results

<u>Experiments on dogs' hindlimb circulation</u>. Carbocromen /CA/ proved to be a drug which continously releases the modulator substance /Szentiványi et al. 1973./. Because of this release the alpha receptors are transformed into beta form; thus they

are not sensitive to the constrictor effect of NA any more
/Fig.1./. The NA dose-response curve /the constrictor effect
on dogs' hind limb circulation/ is shifted to the right after
CA. Propranolol reestablishes the normal state of receptor:
the dose-response curve regains its control position. This
modulation is adrenospecific, it cannot be induced by another
agent, e.g. angiotensin.

The same picture can be obtained when the metabolic level
of the hind limb is elevated by sciatic nerve stimulation, i.
e. the NA dose-response curve is shifted to the right and this
shift can also be prevented by administration of propranolol
/Szentiványi et al. 1970./. A third possibility to obtain this
shift is to administer the modulator substance itself.

/This substance could be demonstrated in coronary sinus
blood of the dog /Szentiványi et al. 1970./. It can be gained
from heart extracts. Extraction was made with pyridin acetate
buffer. The purification ensued on Sephadex G-15 column. The
effective fraction was put on a DEAE cellulose column. All
these steps increased the specific activity. In layer chroma-
tography /BAW system, 0,23-0,24 Rf/ a spot could be identified
with Cl-tollidin staining, the strength of which was parallel
with the activity./

Here again an additional administration of beta blockers
prevents the right shift of the dose-response curve. This
constant release of the modulator substance either by sciatic
nerve stimulation or by carbocromen administration can be
converted into a complete depletion if the stimuli are acting
long enough. So e.g. if the dogs are pretreated for 5-7 days
by 6-10 mg/kg pro die doses of CA, a complete depletion of
the modulator substance takes place. In such a CA-pretreated
dog /Fig. 2./ NA sensitivity does not change after CA. The
beta stimulant ISO evokes only a small effect at high doses.
The diletory effect of 10 µg ISO is as small as that of 0,1µg
ISO on a normal preparation.

Experiments in heart-coronary system.Dog's hind limb is an
organ of lower metabolism thus having a smaller amount of
modulator stored or/and a lower level of synthesis. Hence a
complete depletion of the modulator substance is easy to

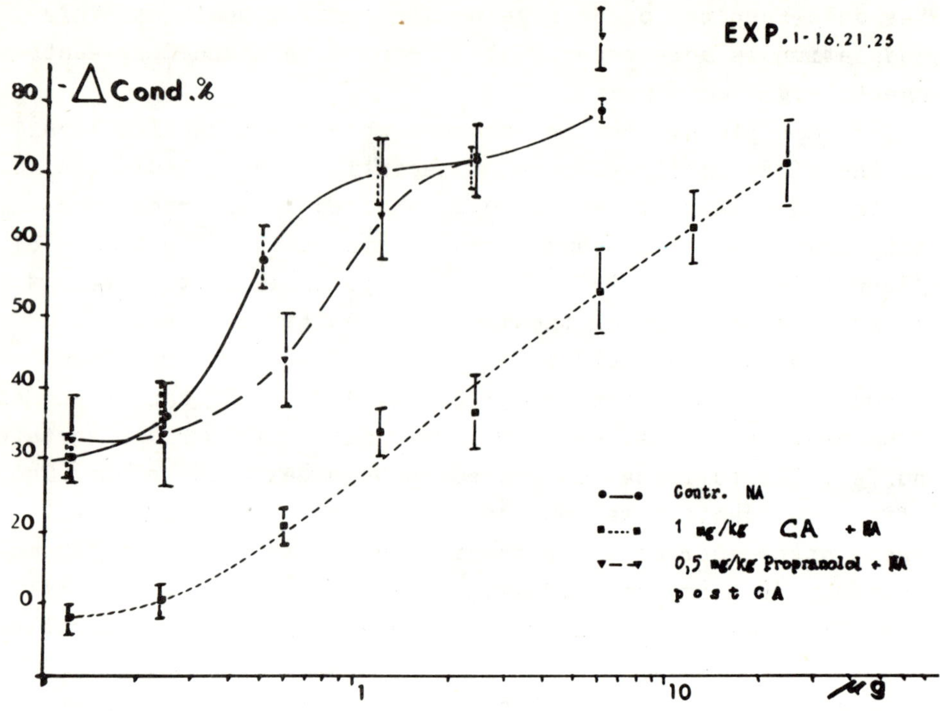

Fig. 1. Dose-response **curve** of NA after CA. Single dots represent mean values as obtained in 18 experiments. Rods: ± standard error of mean. **Ordinate:** - changes in conductivity /%/. Abscisse: NA doses in µg i.a.

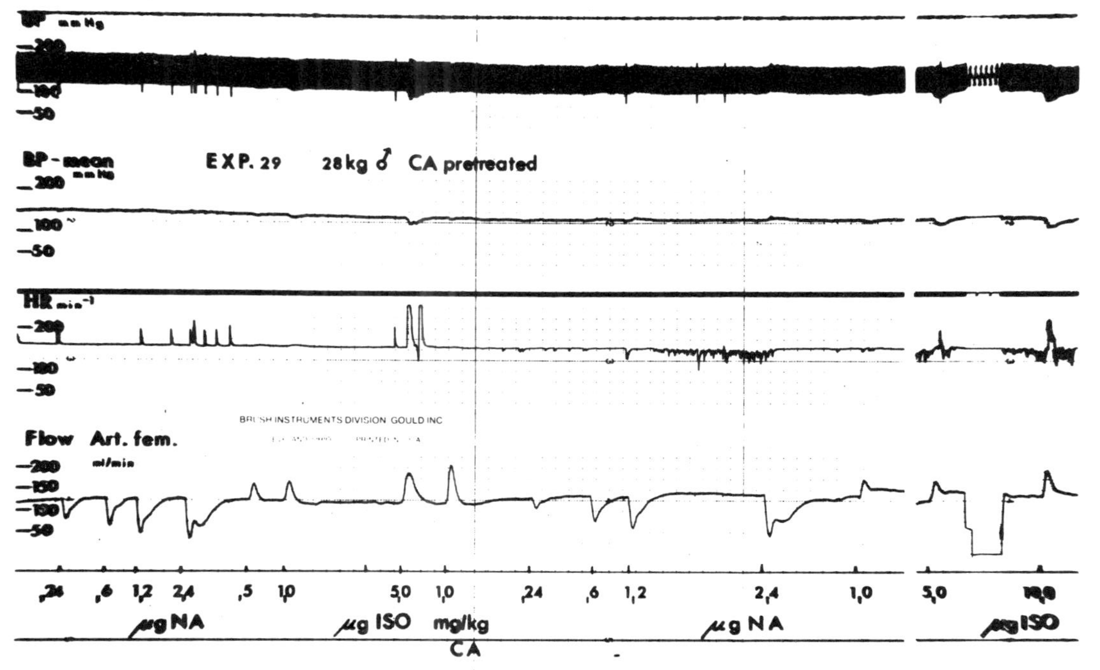

Fig. 2. The adrenergic reactions of a dog pretreated by CA. From top to bottom:
BP: systemic blood pressure; BP mean: mean blood pressure; HR: heart rate;
Flow art. fem.

achieve. Since under such circumstances no metabolic effect
can be done, it can be stated that an alpha to beta transformation is responsible for adrenergic metabolic effect.
Myocardium on the other hand has a much higher metabolic rate
also at rest. To be beta it does not need any exogenic stimulus such as releasing factor or somatic nerve stimulation.
In a resting heart CA increases beta metabolic effect: after
ISO both cardiac contractibility and coronary flow increase.
Hence the same result could be obtained as in the hind limb
preparation: an increase of beta effect.
Now let us see whether a depletion can take place in heart and
coronaries. 17 dogs were pretreated by CA for 5-14 days. The
pretreatment as such did not influence the parameters studied.

Fig. 3. shows that the contractibility of the heart /dp/dt/
does not change after chronic CA pretreatment either when NA
or ISO are administered. From this fact it can be concluded
that modulator is not "stored" but presumably synthesized in
myocardium. Otherwise it could have been depleted. After
chronic CA pretreatment ISO and NA shows a quite different
effect when the coronaries are concerned.

In Fig.4. the changes in enddiastolic coronary resistance
are shown for NA and ISO. It can be seen that in the case of
ISO no change occurs after chronic CA pretreatment /Part B/.
This is quite understandable if we know that ISO is a "pure"
beta stimulant: its cardiac beta metabolic effect is not
changed; beta dilation may also not be altered.

According to the aforementioned modulator theory there are
two possibilities for such a behavior of the ISO effect:

1./ Both myocardium and coronaries possess the modulator
substance /i.e. beta receptors/ and ISO can stimulate both.

2./ The coronaries behave as the hind limb vessels: they
only "store" the modulator substance.
In this second case ISO acting on the modulated myocardial
receptors sets free modulators which are transported to the
coronaries thus making their receptors also beta. If so, NA
which has an alpha constrictor effect too, may exert a smaller
metabolic dilation because NA itself will compete with the
modulator substance on the vascular alpha receptors.

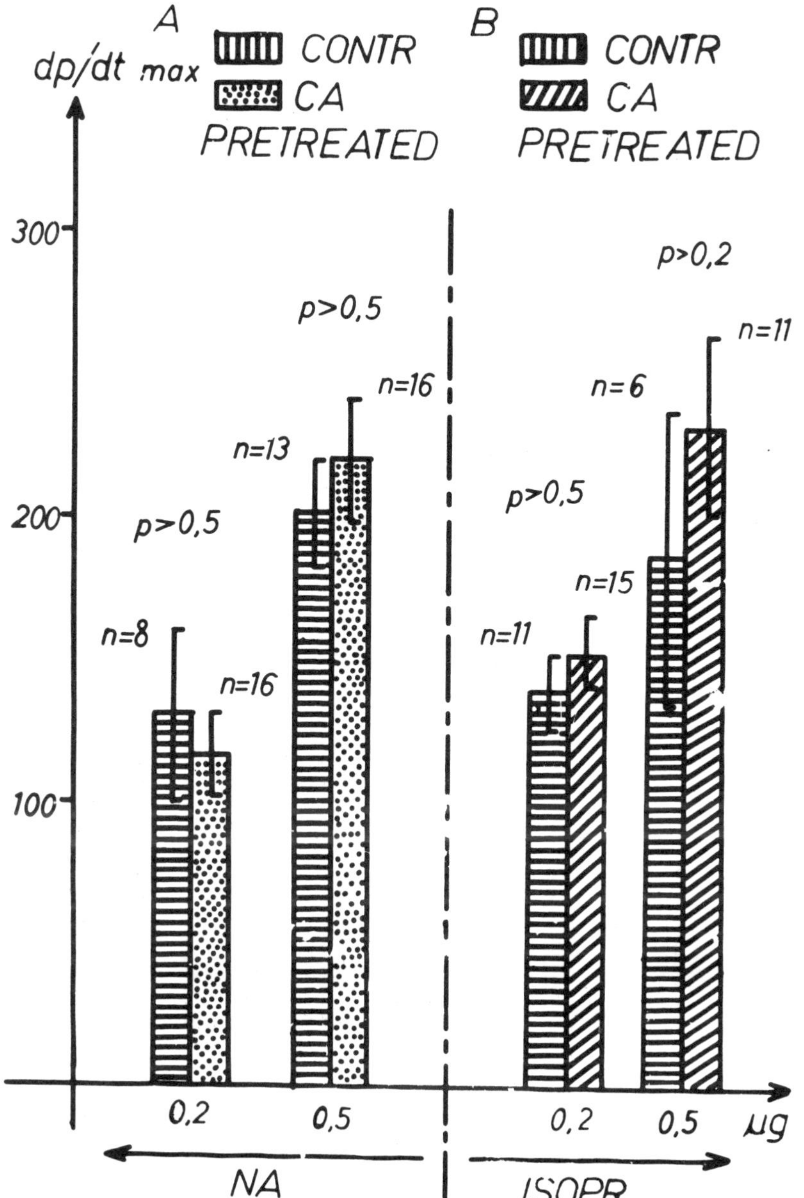

Fig. 3. The effect of NA and ISO on dp/dt max. after CA
pretreatment. Ordinate: dp/dt max. in mmHg/sec.
Abscisse: doses of NA and ISO in µg/kg.

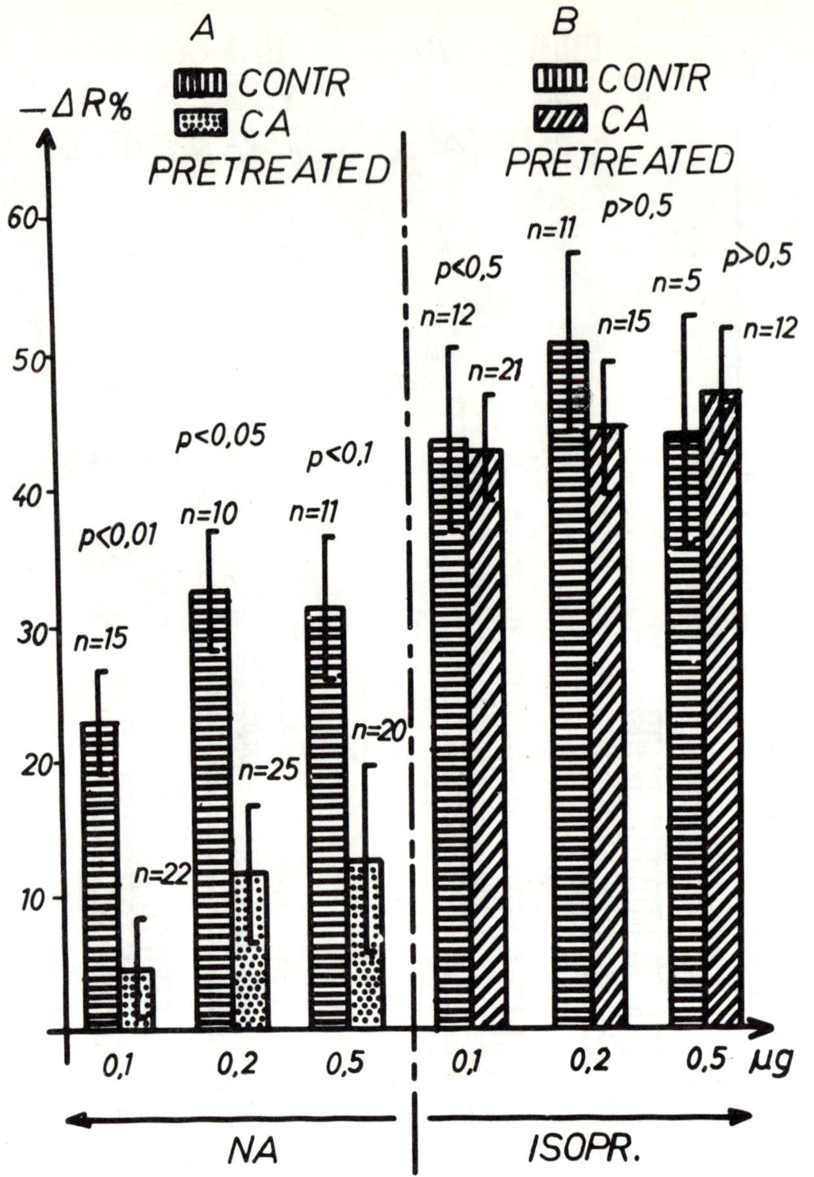

Fig. 4. The changes of the metabolic dilation of NA and ISO after CA pretreatment.
Ordinate: negative changes of EDCR /dilation/ in %
Abscisse: doses of NA and ISO in μg/kg

Fig. 4A. shows that the metabolic dilation to NA is much
smaller in CA pretreated dogs than in the control ones.
Accordingly the constrictor effect /increase in resistance/ to
NA increases after CA pretreatment /Fig. 5A/.
Phenylephrine a more active alpha stimulant causes a more
pronounced increase in resistance after chronic CA pretreatment, although in controls it also has a small dilation /Part
B/. It is worth to note that this constrictor effect may last
for hours! The stronger an alpha stimulant is the longer it
prevents the reattachement of the modulator substance, i.e.
the reestablishing of beta receptors.
The pathological beta modulating effect. Diabetic angiopathy.

What happens if not a correct modulator substance is
synthesized? And if it is synthesized also in areas where it
was previously not present? A pathological form of metabolic
vascular effects may occur. In diabetes even a metabolic
constriction, a beta constriction develops. Aortic spirals of
normal rats respond with contraction to NA. This effect can
be inhibited only by alpha blocking agents. If the aorta is
taken from a diabetic rat the noradrenergic contraction is
abolished by beta blocking agents too /Cseuz et al. 1973./.
If a modulator substance is responsible for this queer effect
it could be only a "false" modulator which is unable for a
full receptor transformation.
The receptor retains its alpha constrictor property but it
can be blocked by beta blocking agents. If this "false" beta
receptor is characteristic to diabetes a beta blocking
substance has to be found which blocks these pathological
beta receptors specifically. We synthesized a substance which
has a similar molecular character as the normal beta blockers
but acts specifically on the diabetic beta receptors. Unlike
Inderal it fails to act on normal beta receptors. The effect
of such a substance is seen in Fig. 6. On the aortic strips
of diabetic rats the constrictor effect of NA is abolished
by NP51. The dose-response curve is shifted to the right by
the drug. The same effect can be seen after Inderal /Cseuz
et al. 1973.; Szentiványi and Pék 1973./. Unlike Inderal NP51

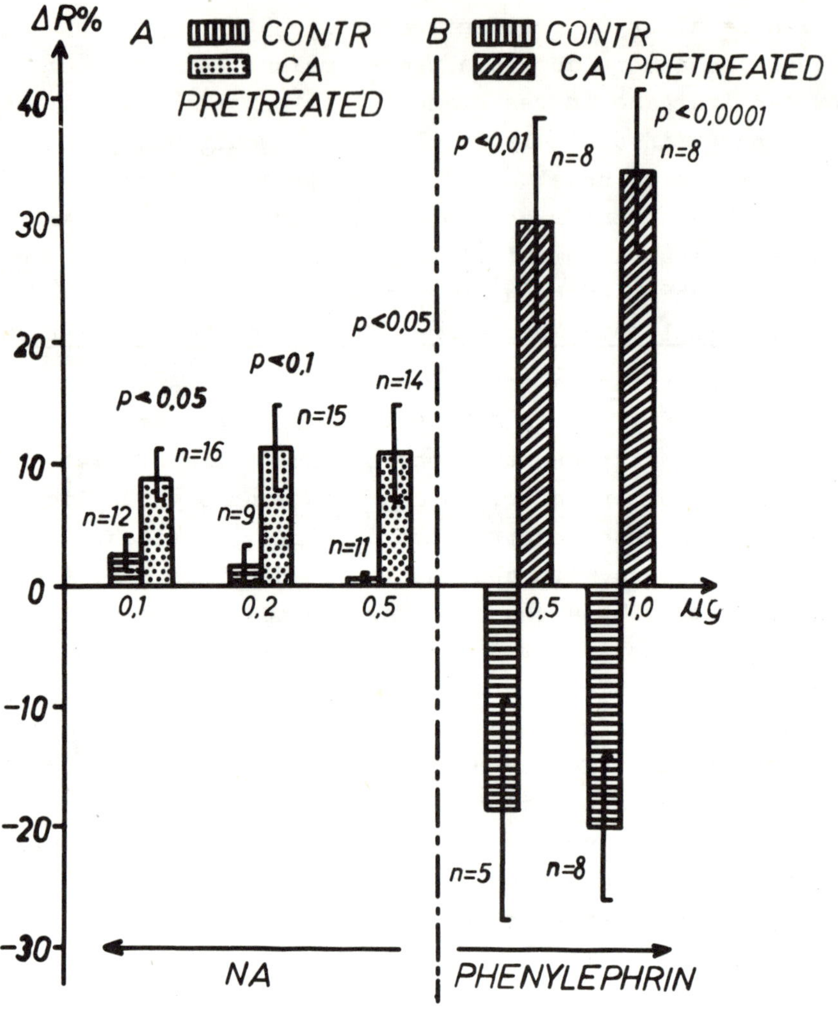

Fig. 5. The constrictor effect of NA and phenylephrine after CA pretreatment.
Ordinate: changes in end-diastolic coronary resistance /EDCR/ in %
Abscisse: doses of NA and phenylephrine in μg/kg

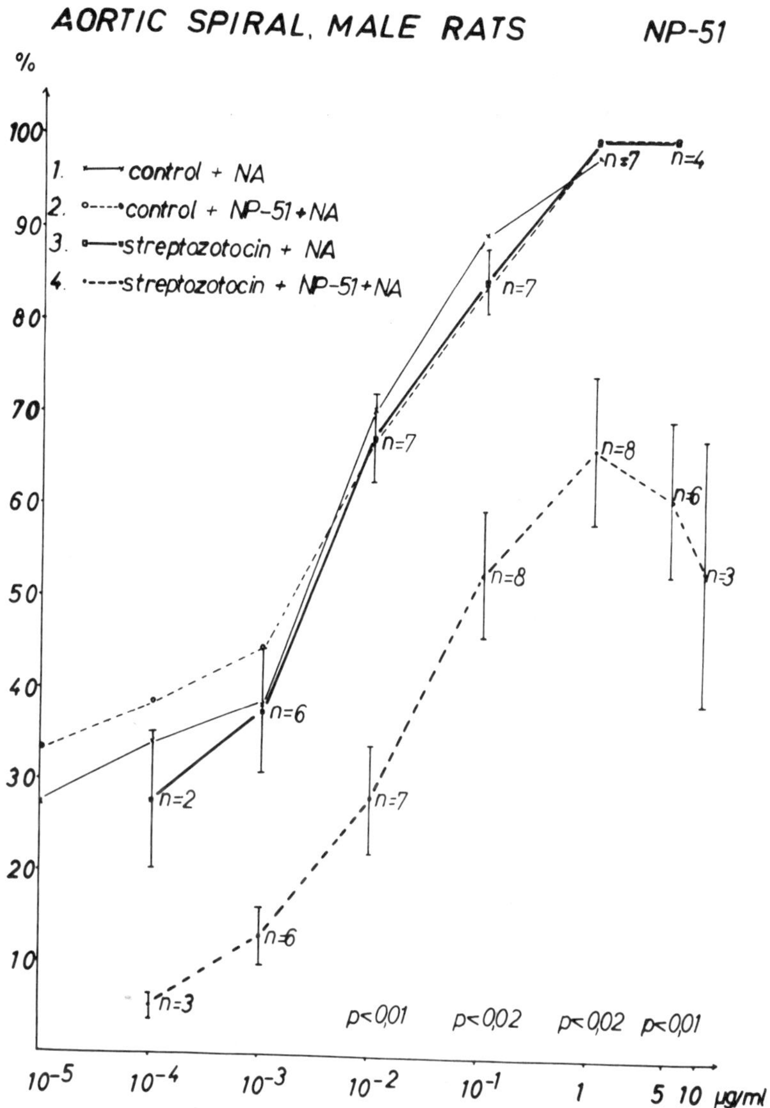

Fig.6. The effect of a specific substance /NP51/ on the
aortic spirals of diabetic and control rats.
Ordinate: the magnitude of NA contractions in percent of the
maximal contraction.
Abscisse: doses of NA in µg/ml

did not **affect** normal beta receptors, i.e. on BP, papillary
muscle, heart rate and on trachea-chain preparation as well
as on the vascular beta receptors it had no effect, when
control animals were concerned.

This action of a specific beta blocker means that a specific
"false" modulator substance is responsible for the false beta
reaction in diabetes.

This above mentioned false beta reaction is the first of the
functional events described in diabetic angiopathy.It develops
in 24 hours after alloxan or streptozotocin treatment. The
last change is the morphological one. The diabetic macro-and
microangiopathy.

It was of general interest whether this first change leads
to the last ones, i.e. to the histological changes. If so, no
matter how many steps are inserted, NP51 has **to** inhibit the
development of diabetic macro-and microangiopathy.
Many of our inbred rats of CFY strain had a latent diabetes
demonstrated by an abnormal elongated glucose tolerance curve.
Some groups of these rats developd spontaneously severe angiopathy: calcium deposition in the great vessels, cartilage
appearance, PAS positivity in the coronaries and aortae,
positive hypoxia staining in the myocardium and vessel walls.
The small vessels and arterioles increased in their diameter
/microangiopathy/. As another sign of microangiopathy the
glomerular membranes were thickened and a PAS positivity of
the glomeruli could be observed.

The membrane **thickening** of the glomeruli could be demonstrated also by electronmicroscopy. All these histological changes
developed in the age of 3-4 months of the animals with latent
diabetes. This could be accentuated by streptozotocin treatment /25 mg/kg-75 mg/kg single dose/.

If the animals with latent diabetes were treated by NP51
/5 mg/kg daily for 3-4 months/ no or very mild histological
changes **could develop.**

This was also the case when the animals were made diabetic
with streptozotocin. In this case streptozotocin administration was followed by an NP51 treatment for 2-3 months.
Fig.7. shows that in the coronaries of diabetic animals the

166

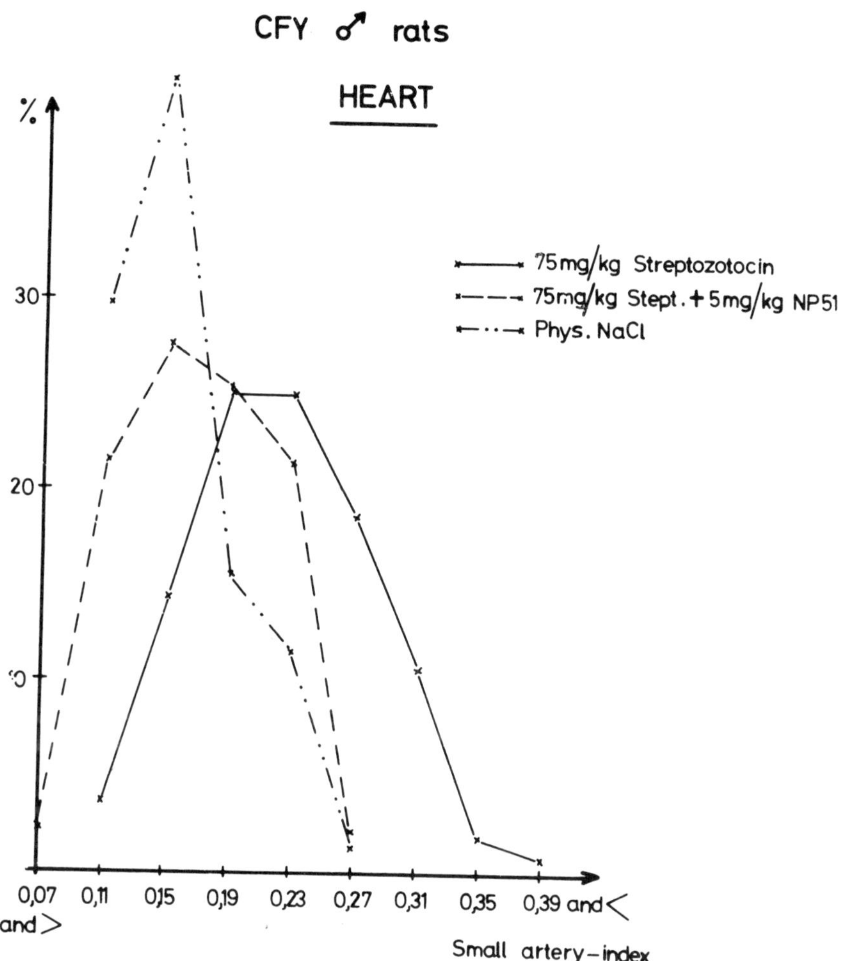

Fig. 7. Changes in wall-thickness of small coronary vessels in diabetes. The effect of NP51 treatment.
Vascular index: wall thickness/diameter of the artery
Abscisse: increasing values of vascular indices
Ordinate: distribution in per cent

diameters of small vessels are shifted to the large values and
how the values of normal wall thickness predominate after NP51
treatment.

Discussion

Rein /1930/ was the first who described that after sciatic
nerve stimulation, i.e. during a metabolic dilation the effect
of adrenalin decreased. On the other hand during metabolic
dilation the alpha receptors are transformed into beta form,
thus unable to respond to alpha stimulant. This transformation
is due to a modulator substance released /Szentiványi et al.
1970.; Szentiványi and Kunos 1969./. Now it is not believed
any more that a stable number, a mixture of alpha and beta
receptors determines the magnitude of an alpha or beta effect
/Ahlquist 1973.; Matheny et al. 1974.: Paradowski 1972./.
The data reported here are in good agreement with the release-
depletion dynamics of this modulator substance /Szentiványi
et al. 1973./.

CA produced on the hindlimb preparation a constant release
of the modulator substance, thus transforming the alpha receptors into beta. Consequently the NA affinity declined, whereas
ISO sensitivity increased. This constant modulator release
could be transformed into depletion by chronic treatment with
CA. Thereafter CA itself failed to produce receptor transformation and a 100-1000 fold decrease in ISO sensitivity ensued.
Since short-lasting sciatic nerve stimulation brings about
the same changes as an acute administration of CA, while long-
lasting stimulation is comparable to CA pretreatment, it could
be concluded that metabolic dilation may be the same or goes
parallel with receptor transformation.

From heart the modulator cannot be depleted thus a continuous synthesis may be conceived. Both ISO and NA effects on
dp/dt were unchanged after CA pretreatment. In coronaries the
depletory function of CA was manifest. While ISO induced the
same dilatory effect as in controls, the noradrenergic
dilation was decreased and the alpha constrictor effect was
pronounced. Both ISO and NA can release modulator substance

168

which supplies also the receptors of the coronaries but
there it is only "stored". ISO releases this "stored" modulator; NA acts also on the not modulated receptor sites thus
causing also constriction. Phenylephrine a "pure" alpha
constrictor agent makes no modulator release from the myocardium and has only a constrictor effect thus showing that
the coronaries were demodulated at least partly. The modulator release from the myocardium fails.

Baron et al. /1972/ showed a more pronounced beta effect on
coronary strips than on those of vessels of striated muscles.
The effect of ISO on the former lasted also longer. According
to the present studies the coronaries get more modulator
substance than the striated muscles.

The fact that the coronaries have the same kind of beta
receptor as myocardium, i.e. beta$_1$ ones /Johansson 1973/,
coincides with the statement that myocardium supplies the
coronaries with modulator substance. It needs no comment that
after beta blockade the alpha constriction of the coronaries
may manifest /Takenaka and Ishinava 1972.; Hashimoto et al.
1960.; Parratt 1965.:Trinker 1973.; Feigl 1967.; Pitt et al.
1967.; Gaal et al. 1966./.

Paradowski /1972/ demonstrated a receptor system in the
brain vessels where beta receptors play a role of a factor
limiting alpha mimetic activity of NA and A. According to his
research a transformation dynamics exists also in cerebral
vessels. Myocardium and brain represent the two most important
areas where metabolic dilation and metabolic autodilation may
play a role.

It is a well known fact that isolation facilitates the
appearance of noradrenergic coronary constriction /Gillis
and Melville 1972./. Under such circumstances the modulator
synthesis diminishes due to a decreased cardiac metabolism
and perhaps to the shock occuring on isolation.

A number of works report on a decrease in beta effect in
acidosis /Schümann et al. 1972.; Marsiglia et al. 1973.; Aus
der Mühlen and Heidenreich 1973 Emerson et al.1974./.
.This could mean that modulator synthesis, which is increased by
elevated metabolism would be stopped when the pH reaches some

value. It is interesting that this pH-induced change in flow
can be blocked by propranolol /Marsiglia et al. 1973./.

According to the presented data there is no reason to speak
about whether the coronaries are innervated by alpha or beta
receptors. Pitt et al./1967/ found a dilatory effect of intracoronary ISO 3-5'' before the starting of cardiac effects. The
metabolic autodilation may have a good answer for such findings.
All the more because coronaries have the same type of beta
receptors as the myocardium. /Johansson 1973./.

That metabolic level plays an important role in receptor
transformation it can be concluded from the actions of
catecholamines in hearts at different temperatures. On amphibian and rat hearts the positive inotropic action of NA could
be blocked by alpha blockers at lower temperatures, while
increasing the temperature the same effect was inhibited by
beta antagonists /Kunos and Szentiványi 1968./. In amphibian
hearts Kunos and Nickerson /1976./ found labelled phenoxybenzamine to be retained at lower temperatures while at higher
temperatures the retaining of labelled propranolol prevailed.

The alpha-beta transformation is dependent also on thyroid
state thus showing how deep a metabolic influence can be
reckoned with /Kunos 1976 /.

All this means that at low temperatures, i.e. metabolic
rates, the receptors lose modulator substance. This happens
also in hypoxia. It was found that NA is an alpha constrictor
agent in the infarcerated zone after coronary ligation
/Grayson et al. 1968.; Vance et al. 1971.; Moore and Parratt
1973./.

Since hypoxia can be effectuated in many instances so e.g.
at high levels of catecholamine release, a mechanism of beta
to alpha transformation may induce further hypoxia and
infarction respectively.

Another use of modulator theory is in diabetic angiopathy.
Here a "false" modulator substance is synthesized unable to
cause a complete alpha-beta receptor transformation. In diabetic vessels constriction to alpha agonists remains unchanged but it can be blocked also by beta antagonists /Cseuz
et al. 1973.; Szentiványi and Pék 1973./.

NP51 is a very weak beta blocker when the normal beta effects
are concerned.On the other hand the diabetic vascular responses
can be equally blocked by Inderal and NP51.Thus NP51 can be
considered as a specific beta blocking agent acting only in
diabetic vessels.

Since specific beta blockers are also effective in diabetic
vessels it can be stated that abnormal beta receptors, i.e.
modulators are produced in the angiopathy.Their selective
blockade may prevent the development of diabetic angiopathy.
NP51 is the first specific drug acting in diabetic vascular
illness.

REFERENCES

Ahlquist,R.P./1973/:Adrenergic receptors:a personal and practic-
    al view.Perspectives in Biology and Medicine.17: 119-122.
Baron,G.D.,Speden,R.N. and Bohr,D.F./1972/:Beta adrenergic re-
    ceptors in coronary and skeletal muscle arteries. Am.J.
    Physiol. 223: 878-881.
Cseuz,R.,Wenger,T.L.,Kunos,G. and Szentiványi,M./1973/:Changes
    of adrenergic reaction pattern in experimental diabetes
    mellitus. Endocrinology 93: 752-755.
Emerson,T.E.jr.,Barker,J.L. and Jelks,G.W./1974/:Effects of
    local acidosis on vascular resistance in dog skeletal muscle.
    Proc. Soc. Exp. Biol. Med. 145: 273-276.
Feigl,E.O./1967/: Sympathetic control of coronary circulation.
    Circ. Res. 20: 262-271.
Gaal,D.G.,Kattus,A.A.,Kolin,A. and Ross,G./1966/: Effects of
    adrenalin and noradrenalin on coronary blood flow before
    and after beta adrenergic blockade.Br.J.Pharm.26: 713-722.
Gillis,Z.A. and Melville,K.J./1972/:Cardiac adrenergic mecha-
    nisms of rabbits with experimentally produced coronary
    atherosclerosis. Atherosclerosis 15: 71-76.
Grayson,J.,Irvine,M.,Parratt,J.R. and Cunningham,J./1968/:
    Vasospastic elements in myocardial infarction following
    coronary occlusion in the dog. Cardiovasc.Res. 2: 54-62.
Hashimoto,K.,Shigei,T.,Imai,S.,Saito,Y.,Yago,N.,Kei,J. and
    Clark,R.E./1960/:Oxygen consumption and coronary vascular
tone in the isolated fibrillating dog heart.A.J.Phys.198:965-970

Johansson,B./1973/: The beta adrenoceptors in the smooth
    muscle of pig coronary arteries. Eur. J. Pharmacol. 24:
    218-224.

Kunos,G./1977/: Thyroid hormone-dependent **interconversion** of
    myocardial alpha-and beta-adrenoceptors in the rat. Br. J.
    Pharmacol. 59: 177-189.

Kunos,G.and Nickerson,M./1976/: Temperature-induced inter-
    conversion of alpha and beta-adrenoceptors in the frog
    heart. J. Physiol./London/ 256: 23-40.

Kunos,G. and Szentiványi, M./1968/: Evidence favouring the
    existence of a single adrenergic receptor. Nature, Lond.
    217: 1077-1078.

Marsiglia,J.C., Cingolani,H.E. and Gonzal**es**,N.C./1973/:
    Relevance of beta receptor blockade to the negative ino-
    tropic effects induced by metabolic acidosis. Cardiovasc.
    Res. 7: 336-343.

Matheny,J.L. and Ahlquist,R.P./1974/: Effects of temperature
    on adrenergic receptors in the iris dilator muscle of
    rabbit. Fed. Proc. 33: 485.

Moore,G.E. and Parratt,J.R. /1973/: Effect of noradrenaline
    and isoprenaline on blood flow in the acutely ischemic
    myocardium. Cardiovasc. Res. 7: 446-457.

Aus der Mühlen,K. und Heidenreich, O. /1973/:Blutdruckwirkung
    von Noradrenalin und Orciprenalin bei erhöhten extra-
    cellulären Wasserstoff - und Calcium- ionkonzentrationen.
    Arch. Int. Pharmacodyn. Ther. 203: 164-174.

Paradowski,A./1972/: Studies on the adrenergic receptor in
    the cerebral circulation. Ann. Med. Sect. Pol. Acad. Sci.
    17: 189-196.

Parratt,J.R./1965/: Blockade of sympathetic beta receptors in
    myocardial circulation. Br. J. Pharmacol. 24: 601-611.

Pitt,B., Elliot,E.C. and Gregg,D.E./1967/:Adrenergic receptor
    activity in the coronary arteries of the unanesthetised
    dog. Circ. Res. 21: 75-84.

Rein,H./1930/: Die Interferenz der vasomotorischen Regulatio-
    nen. Klin. Wochschr. 9: 1485-1489.

Schümann,H.J., Wagner,J. and Reinhardt,D./1972/: Sensitivity
    changes of adrenergic beta-receptors induced by alterations

of metabolic state of isolated organs. Naunyn Schmiedebergs
Arch. Pharmacol. 275: 105-113.

Szentiványi,M., Kunos,G. and Juhász-Nagy,A./1970/: Modulator
theory of adrenergic receptor mechanism: vessels of the
dog hindlimb. Am.J.Physiol. 218: 869-875.

Szentiványi, M. and Kunos, G./1969/: Adrenergic receptive
mechanism in the myocardium and in the coronary vessels.
Symposium Internat. Nancy[*]. pp. 535-539.   [*] Drugs and
metabolism of myocardium and striated muscle.

Szentiványi,M., Nitz,R.E. and Sholtholt,J. /1973/:The effect
of carbocromene on vascular receptors.Naunyn Schmiedebergs
Arch. Pharmacol. Vol. 279 Suppl. pp. 19.

Szentiványi, M. and Pék,L./1973/: Characteristic changes of
vascular adrenergic reactions in diabetes mellitus.
Nature New Biol. 276-277.

Takenaka,F. and Ishinava,T./1972/: Coronary vasomotor responses to the cardiac sympathetic nerve stimulation in the
dog treated with beta adrenoceptor blocking agents. Jap.
J. Pharmacol. 22: 721-723.

Trinker,F.R./1973/: The effect of catecholamines on isolated
perfused coronary arteries of the dog. Arch. Int. Pharmacodyn. Ther. 205: 218-225.

Vance,J.P., Parratt,J.R. and Ledingham,I.M. /1971/:
The effects of hypoxia on myocardial blood flow and oxygen
consumption: negative role of beta adrenoceptors. J. Clin.
Sci. 41: 257-273.

Krieger: Is modulation adreno-specific or can it also be seen
when other vasoconstrictor substances /like angiotensin/ or
vasodilatory substances /like bradykinin, prostaglandins/ are
administered?

Szentiványi: Modulation is adreno-specific, other vasoconstrictor or dilatory substance cannot elicit the phenomenon.
So e.g. sciatic nerve stimulation diminishes both noradrenergic
and angiotensin II-induced vasoconstriction simply by increasing flow, but propranolol reestablishes vasoconstriction only
in the case of NA.

Riemersma: Have you done cross-circulation experiments in which
the depletion of the modulator was examined while the heart was
perfused with blood from separate donor animals?

Szentiványi: We wanted to gather modulator substance in greater
amount. Therefore we used separate dogs for modulator release
and for testing. In order to obtain a greater amount from the
donor dog its stellate was stimulated. The blood of the heart
containing the modulator substance was collected from the coronary sinus. If the acceptor dog's hind limb was perfused with
the sinus blood of the donor, the same effect could be observed
as when the sciatic nerve was stimulated. The constrictor effect of NA was diminished, it reappeared after propranolol. By
this set-up no cross-circulation experiments were needed.

Riemersma: Is the modulator stable?

Szentiványi: After treatment by heat /60°C/ the modulator substance can be deteriorated.

Pogátsa: You stated that NP-51 is active at the very begining
of the diabetic changes, i.e. at the functional level, and it
is doing so in the end state when morphological changes are
also present. What about in the intermediate state?

Szentiványi: We were interested whether preventing the early
functional change may lead to the absence of the late histological ones. The intermediate pathways have not been cleared
yet.

Kunos: I should like to know whether carbocromen has other
side effects that can be blamed for the receptor transformation or anything like.

Szentiványi: The main effects of carbocromen are responsible
for the modulator-like action. It is thought that a constant
modulator release takes place when lower quantities of the
substance are given. Because of increased beta quality the
alpha constrictor effect of NA is diminished after carbocromen,
like during sciatic nerve stimulation, this diminution can be
prevented by propranolol in both cases. In this respect vasodilation to carbocromen may be regarded as a side effect.
There is no relationship between the dilatory effect of carbocromen and its modulator simulating action /i.e. its modulator-
-releasing ability/.

Rubányi: I should like to know whether Ca^{2+} plays any role in
the modulator effect?

Szentiványi: I do not know but Ca^{2+} cannot simulate the modulator effect.

Rubányi: Has modulator substance any role in the Ca^{2+} coupling
effect?

Szentiványi: It has not been proved yet.

THE PROBLEM OF ADRENOCEPTOR-ANTAGONISTS SPECIFICALLY BLOCKING PATHOLOGICALLY TRANSFORMED BETA-ADRENERGIC RECEPTORS

G. P. Leszkovszky and M. Szentiványi

Department of Pharmacology, Chemical and Pharmaceutical Works CHINOIN, Budapest, Hungary

Keeping in mind the interconversion of different adrenergic receptors described for the first time by one of us /Kunos and Szentiványi 1968; Szentiványi et al. 1970/ one has to consider the possibility that, under pathological circumstances, functions due to pharmacological influences on receptors may be qualitatively changed. Things are in fact like this in diabetes mellitus according to recent observations published a few years ago also by one of us: vasoconstriction induced by noradrenaline — a typical alpha-adrenergic effect — in diabetic subjects can be effectively antagonized by beta-receptor blocking agents /Cseuz et al. 1973; Szentiványi and Pék 1973/.

In this case there is a special transformation of adrenergic receptors in diabetes. However, normal beta-blockers acting on these modified receptors at the same time inhibit, of course, other beta-adrenergic reactions in the organism as well. Hence, specificity of diabetic pathologic receptors is pharmacologically confirmed if there are substances influencing exclusively these pathologic adrenoceptors.

In the present paper some compounds of this very type are to be reported on.

It was mentioned in a paper presented at a meeting of the Hungarian Physiological Society a few years ago /Szentiványi et al. 1978/ that contractions induced by noradrenaline in aortic strips of diabetic rats were antagonized also by certain compounds exhibiting some similarities with beta-receptor

blocking agents in their chemical structure. These compounds
were very weak beta-blocking agents as compared to propranolol, having only similarities with it in that the newly
appeared beta-responses could be blocked equally by them and
by propranolol. Unlike propranolol, these substances practically did not affectuate the beta responses of healthy animals, i.e. they affected only the new beta-receptors appeared
in diabetes /Cseuz et al. 1973; Szentiványi and Pék 1973/.

Two of these compounds having the code numbers of NP-18
and NP-51, respectively, have been further studied in detail.

METHODS.

Isolated organs.

Rat aortic strips. Helically cut strips of rat thoracic
aorta were prepared essentially on the basis of the method
of Furchgott and Bhadrakom /1953/. Male rats of the CFY
strain were killed by a blow on the head, the aorta removed
and the strips suspended in an isolated organ bath containing Krebs bicarbonate solution of the following composition
/mmol·liter^{-1}/: NaCl 107.9; KCl 4.7; CaCl$_2$ 2.5; KH$_2$PO$_4$ 1.2;
MgSO$_4$·7H$_2$O 1.2; NaHCO$_3$ 25.0; glucose 6.6. Oxygen was bubbled
through the solution whose temperature was maintained at
37 $^\circ$C. Contractions were recorded by means of an isotonic
lever on a smoked drum. The preparations were allowed to
equilibrate for 3 hours prior to beginning the experiment.
Cumulative dose-response curves to noradrenaline were made
before and after the addition of the appropriate blocking
agent to be studied. Noradrenaline concentrations between
10^{-9} and 5 x 10^{-5} mol·liter^{-1} were used. Responses to noradrenaline were taken for maximal if the last dosis of the
agonist failed to further increase the height of contraction.
Contraction heights were evaluated in per cent terms of maximum responses of that individual preparation recorded in
the absence of any other drug /antagonist/.

Experiments were carried out on aortae from healthy control rats /n = 11/ and animals made diabetic by a single

intravenous injection of 75 mg·kg^{-1} streptozotocin /n = 21/, respectively. Metabolic state of each animal of both control and diabetic groups was checked 2 to 4 days prior to the experiment by blood sugar tests /o-toluidine method, Merkotest^R reagents/ before, and 30, 60 and 120 min after, the intravenous injection of 1 mg·kg^{-1} glucose.

Changes in the noradrenaline effect induced by different blocking agents were evaluated according to Van Rossum et al. /1963/.

<u>Guinea-pig tracheal ring chain preparation</u>. The method of Castillo and de Beer /1947/ was used. Tracheae were taken from guinea-pigs weighing about 300 g and chains were made of about 10 individual cartilage rings. Care was taken to put the membranaceous parts of two adjacent rings always on opposite sides of the chain. The preparation was suspended on an isotonic writing lever under 0.2 to 0.5 g resting tension in a 40 ml organ bath containing Krebs solution /composition see in the preceding paragraph/ maintained at 37 $^\circ$C and vigorously bubbled with pure oxygen. The activity of blocking agents was assessed on the basis of inhibition of relaxation induced by 4 x 10^{-8} mol·liter^{-1} isoprenaline, in per cent terms of the effect of the same isoprenaline concentration in that individual preparation before the addition of any other drug. No drugs increasing spontaneous muscular tone were used throughout the whole experiment.

<u>Cat papillary muscle</u>. Cats of either sex weighing about 2 kg were anaesthetized by sodium pentobarbital /35 mg·kg^{-1} intraperitoneally/. The thorax was opened and the heart quickly excised and put in a Petri dish containing Krebs solution. The right ventricle was opened and one of the papillary muscles or a trabecula was excised together with an appropriate piece of ventricular wall muscle. The excised muscle was attached to bipolar platinium wire electrodes by means of threads previously sutured to the ventricular wall muscle part of the preparation. The free end of the muscle was attached to an isotonic writing lever and the whole preparation was placed in a 10 ml organ bath containing Krebs solution

/composition see above/ maintained at 37° C and vigorously
bubbled with pure oxygen.

The preparation was elclctrically stimulated by square
wave impulses of 1 Hz frequency, 10 msec duration and 1 to
10 V amplitude. The positive inotropic action of noradrenaline added to the organ bath was judged on the basis of increases in the height of contractions. Beta-blocking activities were evaluated as per cent inhibition of the noradrenaline-induced increases in the height of contractions.
Effects of various concentrations are given as mean values
$\pm$ S.E.M. of results obtained in individual preparations.

In vivo experiments.

<u>Chronotropic effects in mice.</u> Influences on the chrono-
tropic responses to i.v. administered isoprenaline were studied in female mice of the CFLP strain weighing about 30 g.
ECG tracings of the animals were recorded under sodium
pentobarbital anaesthesia /100 mg$\cdot$kg^{-1} i.p./ in the IInd
standard lead through intramuscular needle electrodes on an
one-channel ink-writing portable electrocardiograph /O.T.E.
Galileo, Firenze, Italy/ prior to, and 1 min after, the
intravenous injection of 1 µg$\cdot$kg^{-1} isoprenaline. Heart rate
was calculated from R - R distances in the ECG records. Substances to be tested for antagonism to isoprenaline were subcutaneously injected 30 min prior to the latter substance
/i.e. before anaesthesia/. All injectiones to mice were made
in a volume of 0.1 ml per 10 g body weight. Chronotropic
responses i.e. differences between heart rate values recorded
1 min after, and before, isoprenaline, respectively, in various pretreated and control groups were compared by
Student's t test.

<u>Acute haemodynamic effects in cats.</u> Cats of either sex
were anaesthetized by the intraperitoneal injection of 50
mg$\cdot$kg^{-1} chloralose and 300 mg$\cdot$kg^{-1} urethane. The right femoral vein was cannulated for intravenous injections and the
left femoral artery for blood pressure measurement. The
trachea was cannulated and positive pressure artificial

respiration by 13 ml$\cdot$kg^{-1} volume and 16 min^{-1} frequency was
applied. The heart was exposed by a left intercostal thoracotomy and a cannula was transmurally inserted into the left
ventricle /near to the apex of the heart/. Arterial and left
ventricular pressures were measured by means of Elema-Schön-
ander pressure transducers and the latter was electronically
transformed in order to have the dP/dt curve as a measure
of cardiac contractility. All these values and ECG tracings
in the IInd standard lead were recorded on an Elema Mingograf
81 ink-writing polygraph.

Cats were intravenously injected with 0.1 to 0.5 µg$\cdot$kg^{-1}
isoprenaline. The same catecholamine doses were repeated
after the administration of various doses of the substances
to be tested: 0.01 to 1 mg$\cdot$kg^{-1} of propranolol and 1 to 100
mg.kg^{-1} of NP-18 and -51. Inotropic responses were judged on
the basis of per cent changes in the height of the positive
peak of the first derivative of the left ventricular pressure
curve /dP/dt$_{max}$/. Changes in values of single parameters were
tested for significance by Student's paired t test. Only results obtained in those animals showing at the beginning of
the experiment normal positive inotropic responses to isoprenaline were evaluated: cats failing to produce this normal
response were discarded from further studies.

RESULTS

<u>Rat aortic strips.</u> Effects on aortic strips of rats with
streptozotocin-induced diabetes are shown in Fig.1. Cumulative dose-response curves to noradrenaline in the presence of
2 to 3 µmol$\cdot$liter^{-1} concentrations of NP-18 or NP-51 are par-
allelly shifted to the right and at the same time the maximum
heights of the curves are depressed as well. The same effect
is produced by propranolol, too. This effect has been taken
for a dualistic, competitive and non-competitive antagonism
according to Van Rossum et al. /1963/. Therefore both pA$_2$
and pD'$_2$ values for each substance have been calculated:

Substance	pA_2	pD'_2
NP-18	7.00 ± 0.60 /5/	5.06 ± 0.27 /6/
NP-51	6.58 ± 0.27 /6/	5.13 ± 0.16 /8/
Propranolol	6.57 ± 0.43 /7/	5.18 ± 0.16 /8/

In parentheses are given the numbers of individual experiments mean values $\pm$ S.E.M. have been calculated from.

There is no /significant/ difference between correspondent values. Thus, the effects of substances NP-18 and NP-51 on diabetic adrenoceptors are equal to that of propranolol.

No influence on the noradrenaline effect in organs taken from non-diabetic animals is exerted by any of these three substances.

Further experiments were carried out with the aim of comparing these substances in respect to other "normal" beta-receptor blocking activities.

<u>Guinea-pig tracheal ring chains</u>. Antagonism to relaxation induced by isoprenaline was studied in isolated guinea-pig tracheal ring chain preparations /Castillo and de Beer 1947/. The degree of inhibition as a function of drug concentration is shown by Fig.2. Full /100 %/ inhibition is produced by propranolol in concentrations about 1 μmol.liter^{-1} while even 2 to 4 x 10^{-4} mol·liter^{-1} concentrations of both substances NP-18 and NP-51 fail to achieve this effect. Thus, activities of these substances are by nearly three orders of magnitude inferior to that of propranolol in this type of experiment.

<u>Cat papillary muscle</u>. Antagonism to the positive inotropic action of noradrenaline in cat heart papillary muscle is shown in Fig. 3. Curves are here, too, arranged like in the preceding Figure: activities of substances NP-18 and NP-51 are at least by two orders of magnitude inferior to that of propranolol.

Thus, there is a striking difference in experiments in vitro between actions exerted on diabetic pathological adrenoceptors and normal beta-receptors, respectively, by both substances NP-18 and NP-51.

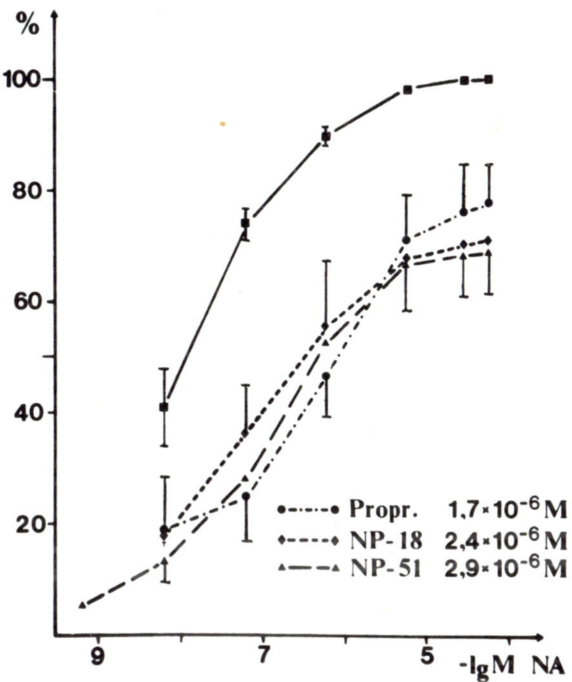

Fig. 1. Cumulative dose-response curves to noradrenaline
of aortic strips of rats with streptozotocin-induced diabetes.
Abscisse: negative logarithm of noradrenaline concentration
/mol.liter^{-1}/. Ordinate: contraction heights in per cent
terms of maximum contractions of individual preparations.
Vertical bars refer to S.E.M. ■: without any antagonist;
●: in the presence of 1.7 μmol·liter^{-1} propranolol;
♦: in the presence of 2.4 μmol·liter^{-1} NP-18; ▲: in the
presence of 2.9 μmol·liter^{-1} NP-51.

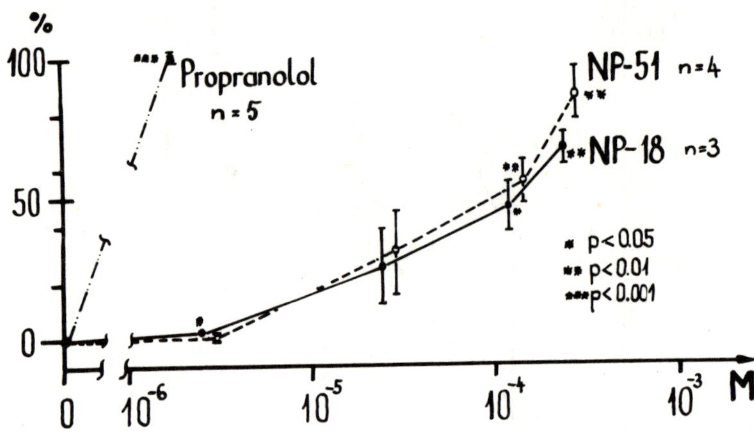

Fig. 2. Inhibition of relaxation induced by isoprenaline /4 x 10^{-8} mol·liter^{-1}/ in guinea-pig tracheal ring chain preparations. Abscisse: concentrations of antagonists /logarithmic scale; mol·liter^{-1}/. Ordinate: differences between relaxation depths recorded without, and in the presence of, the antagonist, respectively; in per cent terms of the original relaxation depth. Vertical bars refer to S.E.M.

■ : propranolol; ● : NP-18; ○ : NP-51.

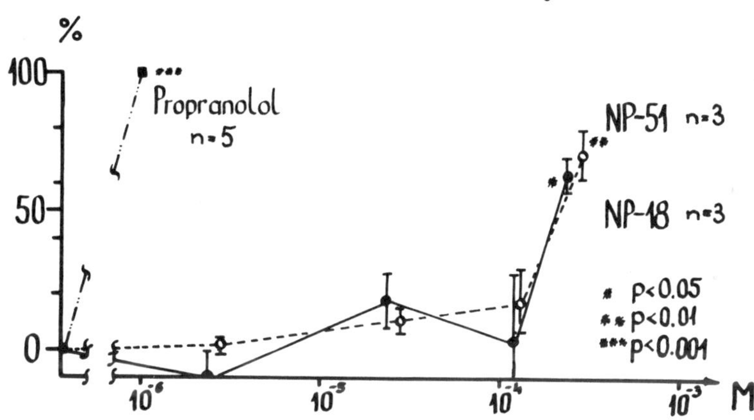

Fig. 3. Inhibition of the positive inotropic action of
noradrenaline /5.9 x 10^{-8} mol·liter^{-1}/ in cat papillary
muscles. Abscisse: concentrations of antagonists /logarithm-
ic scale; mol·liter^{-1}/. Ordinate: differences between increases in contraction amplitudes due to noradrenaline
recorded without, and in the presence of, the antagonist,
respectively; in per cent terms of that increase recorded in
the absence of the antagonist. Vertical bars refer to S.E.M.
■ : propranolol; ●: NP-18; ○ : NP-51.

Also in experiments in vivo there is a similar difference
between actions exerted on normal beta-receptors by substances NP and propranolol, respectively.

<u>Chronotropic effects in mice.</u>As to tachycardia in mice,
due to intravenously injected isoprenaline, no unambigous
inhibition is produced by NP-18 and -51. In Fig. 4. changes
in heart rate induced by 1 $\mu g \cdot kg^{-1}$ isoprenaline in 60 sec
are shown as the function of the doses of drugs administered
subcutaneously 30 min earlier. In these expreiments practolol
was used as an inhibitory drug for comparison. Five $mg \cdot kg^{-1}$
of practolol fully prevented any increase of the heart rate.
NP-18 and NP-51, on the other hand, even in 100 $mg \cdot kg^{-1}$ doses
failed to cause any unambiguous inhibition. Although isoprenaline tachycardia was diminished on higher doses of NP-18 and
after 100 $mg \cdot kg^{-1}$ it was even converted into a decrease in
heart rate, this may be, however, a consequence of the increased basic levels of heart rate after NP-18 as well.
Therefore, the antagonism to isoprenaline may be only
pretensed in this case. NP-51 even in the 100 $mg \cdot kg^{-1}$ dose
did not reduce the chronotropic response to isoprenaline at
all.

<u>Acute haemodynamic effects in cats.</u> In cats under chloral-
ose-urethane anaesthesia acute effects of each substance and
their influences on those of 0.1 to 0.5 $\mu g \cdot kg^{-1}$ isoprenaline
were studied. Some of the data concerning myocardial contractility /dP/dt_{max}/, systolic blood pressure and heart rate
are to be shown in the following Figures.

Left ventricular contractility is considerably decreased
only by 100 $mg \cdot kg^{-1}$ doses of NP-51. /Fig. 5. and 6./. Substance NP-18 in smaller doses shows some trend of a positive
inotropic action both 30 and 60 sec after its intravenous
injection; in 10 $mg \cdot kg^{-1}$ dose it produces a clear, significant
/$p < 0.05$/ positive inotropic effect. NP-51 for its part
exerts in the 10 $mg \cdot kg^{-1}$ dose, both 30 and 60 sec after the
injection, a negative inotropic effect similar to that of
0.01 $mg \cdot kg^{-1}$ propranolol.

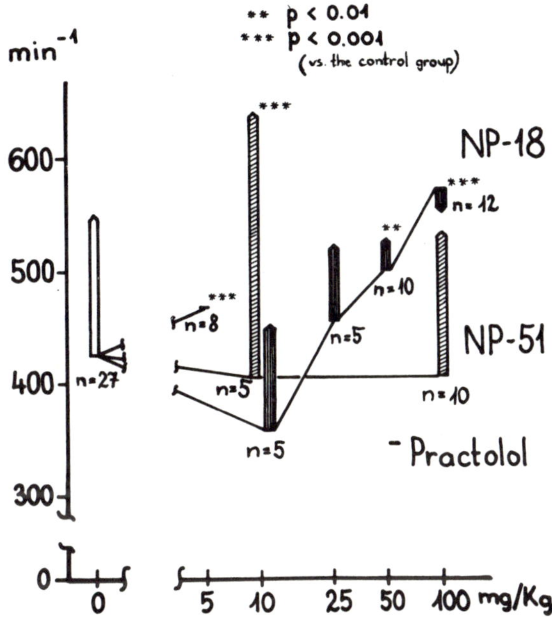

Fig. 4. Changes in heart rate of mice in 60 sec following
the intravenous injection of 1 µg·kg^{-1} isoprenaline. Abscisse: doses of antagonists /logarithmic scale/. Ordinate:
heart rate levels, beats·min^{-1}. The basis of each column
represents heart rate recorded before, and the top that
recorded after, the injection of isoprenaline. Thus, chronotropic responses to isoprenaline in 60 sec are shown by the
heights of the columns. ☐: control mice /no pretreatment/;
■: practolol; ▦: NP-18; ▨: NP-51.

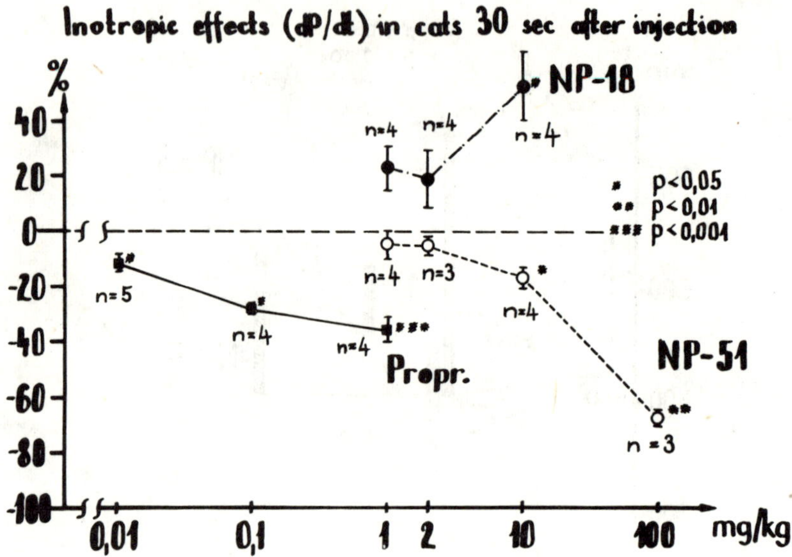

Fig. 5. Inotropic effects recorded in cats under chloralose-urethane anaesthesia 30 sec after the intravenous injection. Abscisse: doses /logarithmic scale/. Ordinate:
changes in the mm height of the positive peak of the dP/dt
curve i.e. of the first derivative of the left ventricular
pressure, in per cent of the original /pre-injection/ level.
Vertical bars refer to S.E.M.

■ : propranolol; ● : NP-18; ○ : NP-51.

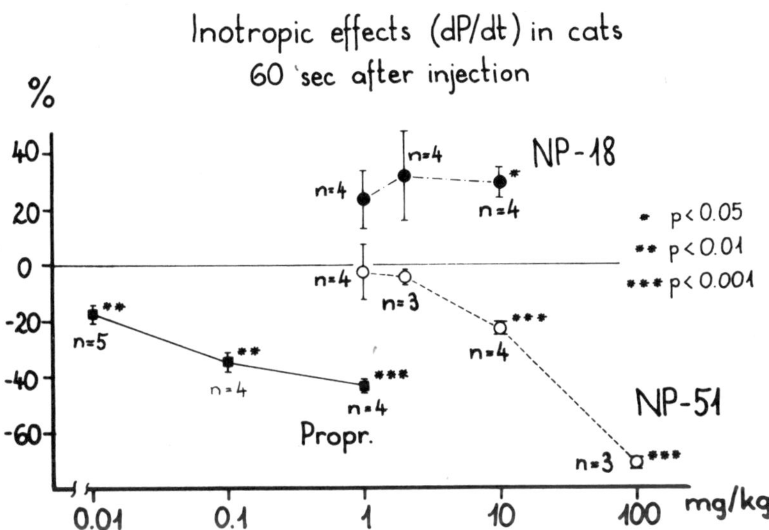

Fig. 6. Inotropic effects recorded in cats under chloralose-urethane anaesthesia 60 sec after the intravenous injection. Abscisse: doses /logarithmic scale/. Ordinate:
changes in the mm height of the positive peak of the dP/dt
curve i.e. of the first derivative of the left ventricular
pressure, in per cent of the original /pre-injection/ level.
Vertical bars refer to S.E.M.

■ : propranolol;　● : NP-18;　○ : NP-51.

As to systolic blood pressure /Fig. 7./, dose-response curves to both substances NP-18 and NP-51 are very similar. They are shifted by about two to three orders of magnitude to the right from that to propranolol. Their effect cannot be regarded as considerable in doses smaller than 100 $\text{mg} \cdot \text{kg}^{-1}$.

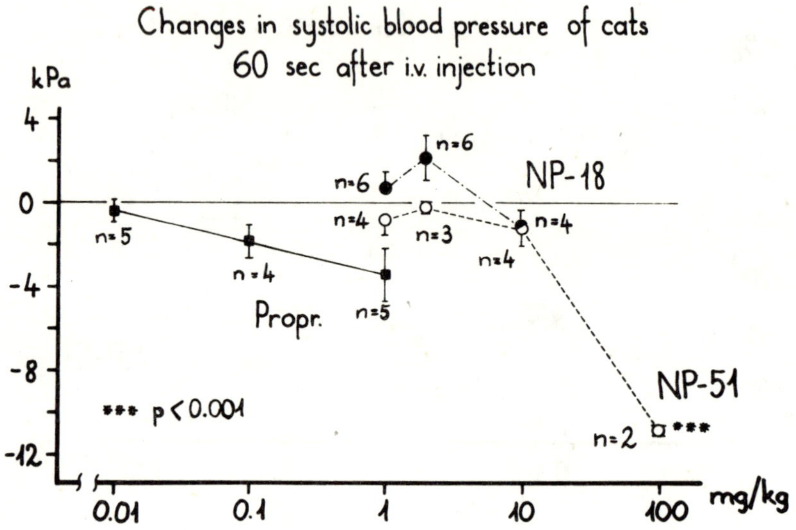

Fig. 7. Changes in systolic blood pressure of cats under chloralose-urethane anaesthesia in 60 sec following the intravenous injection. Abscisse: doses /logarithmic scale/. Ordinate: differences between systolic blood pressure levels /kPa/ recorded 60 sec after, and prior to, the injection. Vertical bars refer to S.E.M.
■ : propranolol; ● : NP-18; o : NP-51.
Conversion: 1 kPa ≃ 7.5 mm Hg.

190

Things are like this also from the point of view of heart
rate as summarized in the next Figure /Fig. 8./.

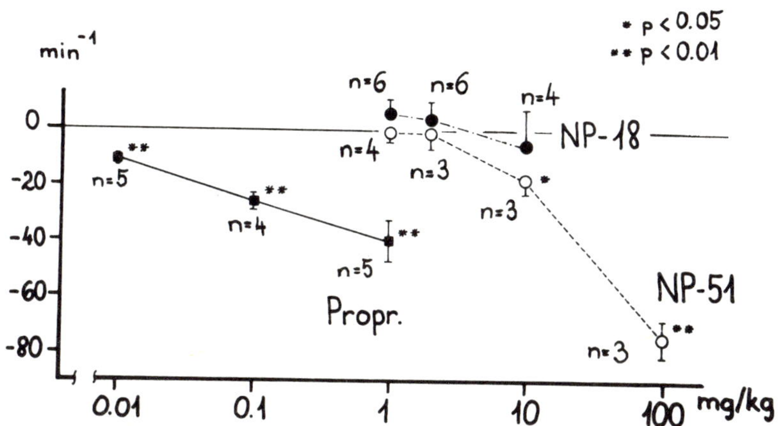

Fig. 8. Chronotropic effects in cats under chloralose-
-urethane anaesthesia 60 sec after the intravenous injection.
Abscisse: doses /logarithmic scale/. Ordinate: differences
between heart rates /beats·min^{-1}/ recorded 60 sec after, and
prior to, the injection. Vertical bars refer to S.E.M.
■ : propranolol; ● : NP-18; ○ : NP-51.

The positive inotropic action of isoprenaline is not considerably diminished by substances NP-18 and -51 /Fig.9./.
NP-18 rather potentiates increases in contractility induced
by isoprenaline. At the same time positive inotropic responses to isoprenaline are inhibited by doses of propranolol 100
to 1000 times lower than those of substances NP-18 and NP-51.

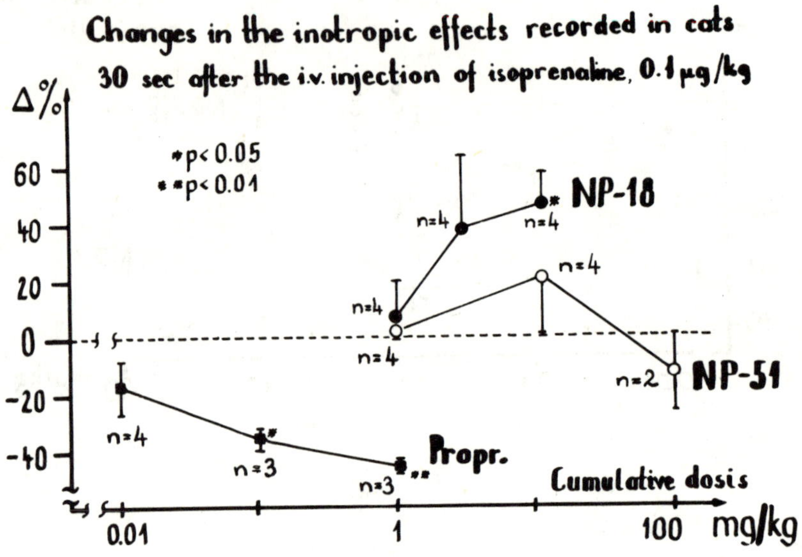

Fig. 9. Changes in the inotropic responses to 0.1 µg·kg^{-1}
isoprenaline recorded 30 sec after its injection. Abscisse:
cumulative doses of antagonists /logarithmic scale/.
Ordinate: differences between isoprenaline-induced per cent
increases of the positive peak of the dP/dt curve i.e. of
the first derivative of the left ventricular pressure after,
and before, antagonist administration, respectively. Vertical
bars refer to S.E.M.

■ : propranolol; ● : NP-18;   ○ : NP-51.

As to systolic blood pressure, reduction of hypotensive
responses to isoprenaline is plotted as a function of doses
/Fig. 10./. A trend of some inhibition proportional to doses
may be observed in the case of NP-51 but even this trend, if
accepted at all, is at least some 100 times weaker than the
effect of propranolol. NP-18 in this respect devoids any such
activity.

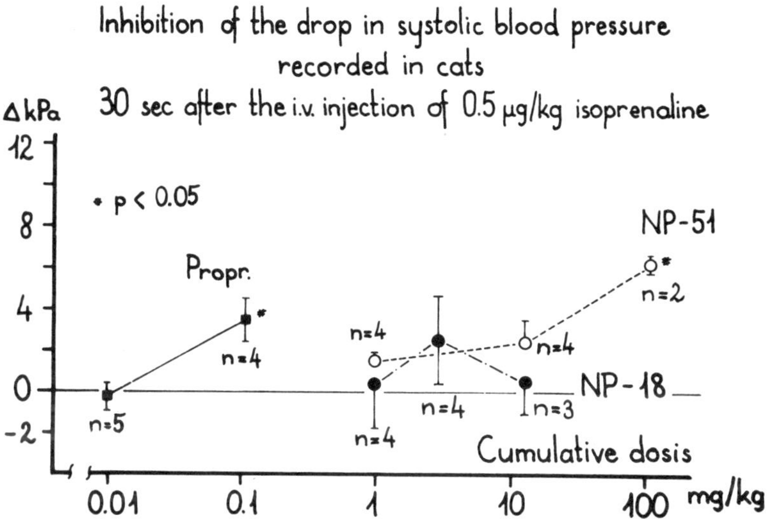

Fig. 10. Inhibition of the drop in systolic blood pressure
recorded in cats under chloralose-urethane anaesthesia in 30
sec after the intravenous injection of 0.5 µg·kg^{-1} isoprenaline. Abscisse: cumulative doses of antagonists /logarithmic
scale/. Ordinate: differences between changes in systolic
blood pressure /kPa/ induced by isoprenaline in 30 sec after,
and before, antagonist administration, respectively. Vertical
bars refer to S.E.M. ■ : propranolol; ● : NP-18; ○ : NP-51.
Conversion: 1 kPa ≃ 7.5 mm Hg.

In contrast to propranolol, the positive chronotropic
action of isoprenaline /Fig. 11./ is left unaffected by even
high doses of NP-18 and NP-51.

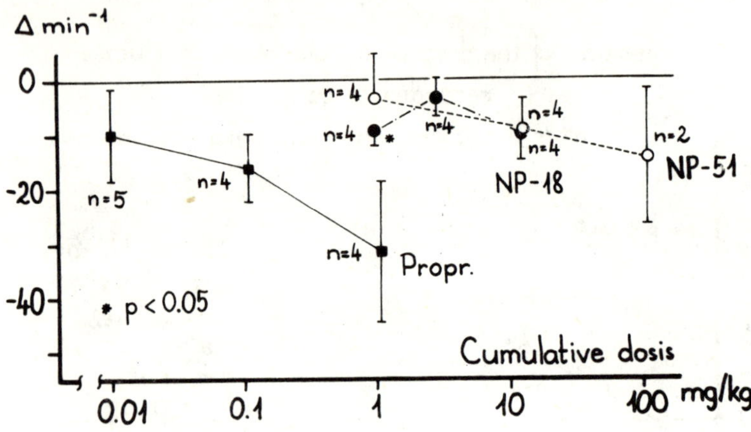

Fig. 11. Changes in chronotropic effects recorded in cats
under chloralose-urethane anaesthesia in 15 sec after the
intravenous injection of 0.1 μg·kg^{-1} isoprenaline. Abscisse:
cumulative doses of antagonists /logarithmic scale/. Ordinate: differences between increases in heart rate /beats·min^{-1}/
induced by isoprenaline after, and prior to, antagonist administration, respectively. Vertical bars refer to S.E.M.
■ : propranolol; ● : NP-18; ○ : NP-51.

DISCUSSION

It is clear from both in vitro and in vivo experiments
that pathological receptors in diabetic animals' blood vessels
are specifically affected by substances NP-18 and NP-51. These
receptors are blocked by them like by propranolol while their
influence on "normal" beta-adrenergic receptors is at least
some 100 to 1000 times inferior to that of propranolol.

It has to be emphasized that the same pattern of pharmacological activity is shared by two — structurally somewhat related — distinct chemical substances. Thus, this pattern cannot
be regarded as a **fortuitous phenomenon** but so much the more
as evidence supporting pharmacological specificity of newly
formed diabetic pathological adrenoceptors.

This specificity seems to be a pathological development of
normal receptor quality. It may be supposed that synthesis of
a "false" modulator substance of pathological structure is
responsible for this specificity. Therefore alpha-receptors
involved in vascular smooth muscle contractions may become
sensitive to beta-adrenoceptor blocking agents.

This change in adrenergic receptor reactivity seems to be
the first step in that pathological mechanism producing at
last the manifestation of diabetic angiopathy. All links of
this process are, of course, not fully made clear. An un-
answered question is e.g. the role of insulin receptors: what
connection do they have with changes in reactivity of adrenergic receptors? Perhaps, an antagonism may be present at the
level of receptors, too.

In any case, we are of the opinion that these substances
having been shortly reported on and similar compounds are by
all means worthy of serious attention. From the theoretical
point of view they do contribute to the evidence supporting
the existence of certain specific pathological adrenergic
receptors. From the practical point of view their further investigation seems to be indicated with the aim — and hope —
of developing new drugs effective against diabetic angiopathy,
the result of a long series of events the first of which is

the specific alteration of reactivity of adrenergic receptors
effectively and specifically influenced by such compounds.

REFERENCES

Castillo, J.C., de Beer, E.J. /1947/: The tracheal chain. I.
    A preparation for the study of antispasmodics with partic-
    ular reference for bronchodilator drugs.
    J.Pharmacol.Exp.Ther. 90: 104-109.
Cseuz, R., Wenger, Th.L., Kunos, G., Szentiványi, M. /1973/:
    Changes of adrenergic reaction pattern in experimental
    diabetes mellitus. Endocrinology, 93: 752-755.
Furchgott, R.F., Bhadrakom, S. /1953/: Reactions of strips of
    rabbit aorta to epinephrine, isopropylarterenol, sodium
    nitrite and other drugs. J.Pharmacol.Exp.Ther.108: 129-143.
Kunos, G., Szentiványi, M. /1968/: Evidence favouring the
    existence of a single adrenergic receptor.
    Nature, 183: 1077-1078.
Szentiványi, M., Faragó, I., Miklya, Ildikó, Takács, K.
    /1978/: Experimental model and therapeutic responsiveness
    of diabetic angiopathy./Abstracts of the lectures deliv-
    ered at the 42nd Congress of the Hungarian Physiological
    Society, June 10-12, 1976./
    Acta physiol.Acad.Sci.Hung. 51: 195-196.
Szentiványi, M., Kunos, G., Juhász-Nagy, A. /1970/:
    Modulator theory of adrenergic receptor mechanism:
    vessels of the dog hindlimb. Am.J.Physiol. 218: 869-875.
Szentiványi, M., Pék, L. /1973/: Characteristic changes of
    vascular adrenergic reactions in diabetes mellitus.
    Nature New Biology, 244: 276-277.
Van Rossum, J.M., Hurkmans, J.A.Th.M., Wolters, C.J.J. /1963/:
    Cumulative dose-response curves. II. Technique for the
    making of dose-response curves in isolated organs and the
    evaluation of drug parameters.
    Arch.int.Pharmacodyn.Ther. 143: 299-330.

DISCUSSION

<u>Kunos</u>: Did you make any study on d-propranolol, too, in
order to show that the beta potency of the drug is responsible
for the mentioned effects?

<u>Leszkovszky</u>: In the main drift of the experiments Inderal
ampoules of I.C.I. were used. On the other hand, not only
propranolol but also other beta blockers were administered.
They were equally effective as propranolol.

<u>Kunos</u>: Are there any other non-adrenergic /blood pressure,
heart rate etc./ effects which can be blocked by NP-51?

<u>Leszkovszky</u>: No, the drug is specific. As I pointed out,
it is a very weak beta blocker in normal preparations.

<u>Mattsson</u>: Could you, please, inform me about the chemical
structure of NP-51?

<u>Leszkovszky</u>: Here I give you the structural formula of
NP-51:

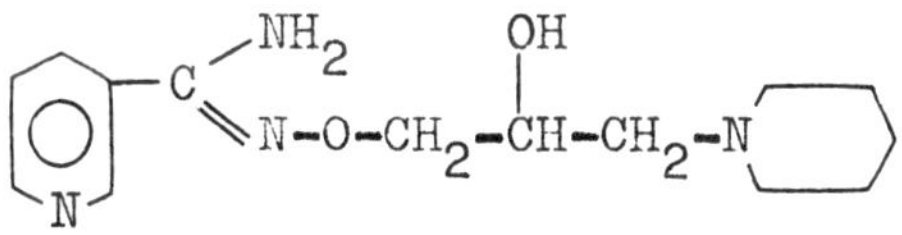

$$\text{pyridine-}C\!\!\begin{array}{c}NH_2\\ \diagdown\\ N-O-CH_2-CH(OH)-CH_2-N\text{(piperidine)}\end{array}$$

A HISTOLOGICAL STUDY OF EXPERIMENTAL DIABETIC ANGIOPATHY

Cs. Vértesi and M. Szentiványi
Department of Pharmacology, Chemical and Pharmaceutical Works CHINOIN, Budapest, Hungary

It is well known that both in human and experimental diabetes macro-and microangiopathies manifest. It was assumed that diabetic disfunction of the vessels may lead to these morphological changes./Szentiványi and Pék 1973; Cseuz et al. 1973/. It has been shown that some beta blocking substances are able to inhibit this pathological function. The aim of the present work is to elucidate whether the finally developed morphological disorders can be prevented by the blockade of these early functional changes.

METHODS

The experiments were done in an inbred strain of CFY rats. Blood sugar curves showed latent diabetes in some of the members of this group, probably because of the inbreeding. If spontaneous diabetes was present it could be aggravated by streptozotocin treatment. Each animal was given 75 mg/kg streptozotocin in a single intravenous injection. This was found the most appropriate dose for the drug. NP51 was administered for 4 months in a 5 mg/kg/day dose. The experiments were carried out on males weighing 250-300 g. The material being studied consisted of a non-diabetic control group, of a group in which streptozotocin had been administered. In a third group streptozotocin and also NP51 had been administered. The negative control group involved also Long-Evans rats, which did not have latent diabetes. Each group contained 10-10 animals. After the administration period the animals were killed and the viscera were removed for histological studies.

Studies were carried out on the coronaries and myocardium with
its capillary tree, as well as in the aorta, femoral artery and
on the complete renal vascular bed.

The studies were performed mainly by light microscopy, but
in some cases, when basal membranes of the glomeruli were
examined an electron microscopic study was also added. The
slices were elaborated by stainings of Haemalaun-eosin,
PAS-Hale, ABT, van Gieson, Gömöri silver-impregnation and a
specific hypoxia staining method elaborated by us was also
used /Vértesi and Szentiványi 1976/. This latter staining
for hypoxic events consists of the following steps:

1./ Remove paraffin with alcohol and distilled water.
2./ Treat with Solution "A", 2 min.
3./ Rinse in distilled water.
4./ Treat with Solution "B", 2 min.
5./ Rinse in distilled water.
6./ Differentiate in Solution "A", 1 min.
7./ Wash repeatedly in tap-water, 10 min.
8./ Rinse in distilled water.
9./ Dehydrate in alcohol, clear in xylene, mount in balsam.

Solution "A": Ferriammonium sulphate   3 g
              /Violet crystals/
              Distilled water   97 g

Solution "B": Hematoxylin   0,5 g
              Alcohol 96 per cent   5,0 g
              Distilled water   95,0 g
              Mercury oxide /II/   0,5 g

By means of this staining a blueish-black color develops in
the hypoxic areas. This was proved by local ligation of
several vessels as well as in general hypoxia /Vértesi and
Szentiványi 1976/. In the quantitative studies serial sections
of various vessels were evaluated. In these cases at least
100 vascular indices were determined.

It has been shown that mainly the thickening of the media
is characteristic of diabetes, therefore a vascular index was
used in this respect.

Vascular index= media thickness/diameter between the two
lamina elastica externa.
The   vascular indices were grouped in % distribution.

RESULTS

Figure 1. shows how the "total" vascular bed /coronaries,
mesenterium, kidneys/ behaves in diabetes, in the control
group and in the one where also NP51 was administered. A
shift of the diabetic curve towards the vessels of thicker
vascular walls, i.e. greater vascular index numbers can be
seen. After NP51 pretreatment a shift to normal values of
the index numbers is effectuated. Thus an increase in the
number of the vessels of narrower walls is manifest, while
a drop in that of the thicker vessels is present. In order to
evaluate how far the single vascular beds are involved a
comparison with each other was also important.
Figure 2. shows a shifting to greater values of the vascular
indices in diabetic mesenteric vessels.

The vascular indices of the kidneys are presented in Fig.3.
A similar shift of the values can be seen as in the former
Fig.

Fig.4. shows a diabetic coronary vessel with Hemalaun-
eosin staining. A thickening of the vessel wall is demonstrated. NP51 pretreatment inhibits this thickening of
the vessel wall. In Fig. 5. no thickening of the wall is
present. This animal was treated for 4 months by NP51 after
making it diabetic.

As another histological feature of the diabetic vessels a
mucopolysaccharide accumulation can be observed.

An increased quantity of neutral and acidic mucopolysaccharides is present in the diabetic animals. PAS positivity in
coronary vessels increases pathologically. When the animal
was treated by NP51 no change in the mucopolysaccharide
content was manifest.

Also hypoxia takes place in the diabetic vessels.

It is pronounced also in the parenchymatous cells.By our
specific staining patchy dark areas characterize hypoxic
involvement. Fig. 6. shows that the myocardium of a diabetic
animal is really hypoxic. If the animals were pretreated by
NP51 no hypoxic changes could be observed in the myocardium
of the diabetic animals./Fig. 7./
Electronmicrograms of diabetic animals show a thickening of
the basal membrane of the glomeruli /Fig. 8./. This can be
prevented by NP51. /Fig. 9./

DISCUSSION

It is well known that a macro-and microangiopathy develops in
diabetes.The latter manifests mainly in the kidney-vessels.The
characteristic changes are described in details by Mincu /1975/
and by Colwell /1975/.The main histological events are the PAS
positivity of accumulated neutral mucopolysaccharides as well
as a thickening of the basal membrane of the glomeruli.A number
of authors deal with the organic changes of the basal membranes
in histochemical and electronmicroscopic studies, respectively.
/Farquhar and Hopper, 1951;Lazarow and Speidel, 1964;Bloodworth
1965;Berkman and Rifkin, 1966;Ireland and Patnaik, 1967;
Beisswenger and Spiro, 1970; Spiro, 1971;Siperstein and Raskin,
1973; Mincu, 1975/.
The same changes could be observed also in the present
studies. Almost all micro-and macroangiopathic changes of
diabetic rats could be prevented in the present experiments.
Perhaps the most intriguing event that occurs in diabetes is
the hypoxia in myocardium as well as that in the media of
several vessels. This may be the cause of other changes, and
may be the consequence of incomplete substrate oxygenation.
Our method indicating hypoxia is very sensitive. In rats a
few minutes after ligation of the coronaries a positive reaction
could be observed. Another early manifestation of diabetic
angiopathy is mucopolysaccharide deposition. Both changes were
inhibited by NP51 treatment. As a final stage of diabetic
smooth muscle anomalies the appearance of cartilage can be

mentioned. No appearance of cartilage was present in animals
treated by NP51. It can be concluded that early functional
changes lead to the latest histological ones:
by inhibiting the formers the latters cannot develop.

REFERENCES

Beisswenger, P.J., Spiro, R.G. /1970/: Human glomerular
    basement membrane: chemical alteration in diabetes melli-
    tus. Science 168: 596-598.
Berkman,J., Rifkin,H. /1966/: New aspects of diabetic micro-
    angiopathy. Ann. Rev. Med. 17: 83-91.
Bloodworth,J.M.B., Jr. /1965/:Experimental diabetic glomerulo-
    sclerosis II. The dog. Arch. Pathol. 79: 113-125.
Bradley, R.F. /1971/: Coronary artery disease.
    In:Fajans,S., and Sussmann,K.: Diabetes Mellitus:Diagnosis
    and Treatment. New York. American Diabetes Association
    Inc. 1971. vol. III. pp. 295-303.
Colwell, J.A.: Clinical recognition and treatment of diabetic
    vascular disease. 1975. Charles C. Thomas Publisher U.S.A.
Cseuz,R., Wenger,T.L., Kunos,G. and Szentiványi, M. /1973/:
    Changes of adrenergic reaction pattern in experimental
    diabetes mellitus. Endocrinology 93: 752-755.
Farquhar,M.G., Hopper,J. /1951/:Diabetic glomerulosclerosis:
    electron and light microscopic studies. Am.J.Path. 35:
    721-754.
Ireland,J.T., Patnaik,B.K. /1967/: Glomerular ultrastructure
    in secondary diabetics and normal subjects. Diabetes 16:
    628-635.
Kimmelstiel,P., Osawa,G. /1966/: Glomerular basement membrane
    in diabetes. Amer. J. Clin. Pathol. 45: 21-31.
Lazarow,A., Speidel,E. /1964/: The chemical composition of
    the glomerular basement membrane and its relationship to
    the production of diabetic complications.
    In: Siperstein,M.D.,Colwell,A.R. and Meyer,K. /Eds./:
    Small blood vessel involvement in diabetes mellitus.
    Washington,D.C., American Institute of Biological Sciences
    1964. p. 127.

Mincu,M.: Diabetic macro-and microangiopathy. Gruyter, Berlin 1975.

Siperstein,M.D., Raskin,P., /1973/: Electron microscopic quantification of diabetic microangiopathy. Diabetes 22: 514-524.

Spiro,R.G. /1963/: Glycoproteins and diabetes. Diabetes 12: 223-231.

Spiro,R.G. /1967/: Studies on the renal glomerular basement membrane. Preparation and chemical composition. J. Biol. Chem. 242: 1915-1922.

Spiro,R.G. /1971/: Glycoproteins-Diabetic Microangiopathy. In: Marble,A., White,P., Joslins Diabetes Mellitus, 11 ed. Philadelphia, Lea and Febiger 1971, p. 146.

Vértesi, Cs. and Szentiványi, M. /1976/: A new staining method for hypoxic changes with special reference in atherosclerosis. II. Hungarian Arteriosclerosis Conference, Budapest.

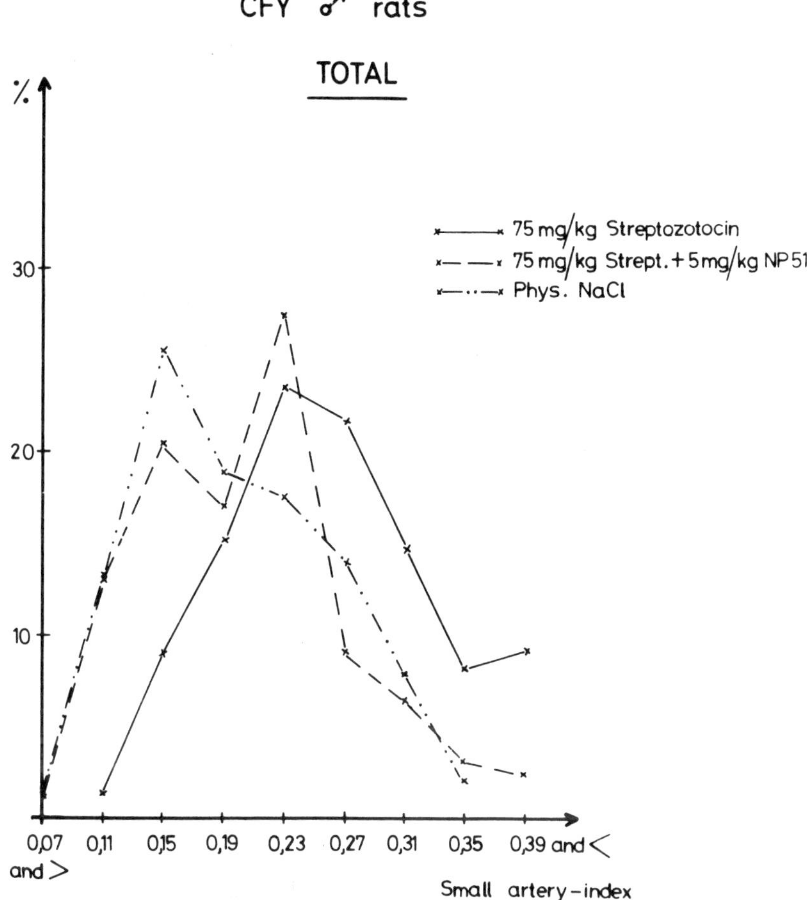

Fig. 1. Vascular-index changes in diabetes.
   Abscisse: values of arterial indices.
   Ordinate: % distribution of the values. /Coronaries,
         mesenteric and renal arteries./

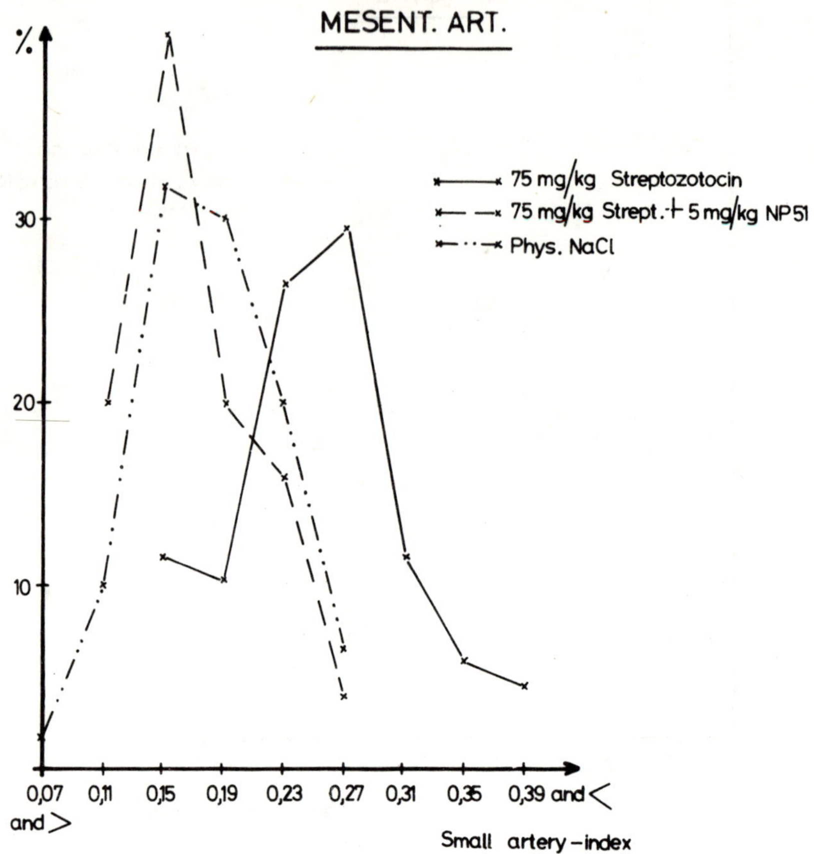

Fig. 2. Vascular-indices in the mesenteric arteries.
See fig. 1.

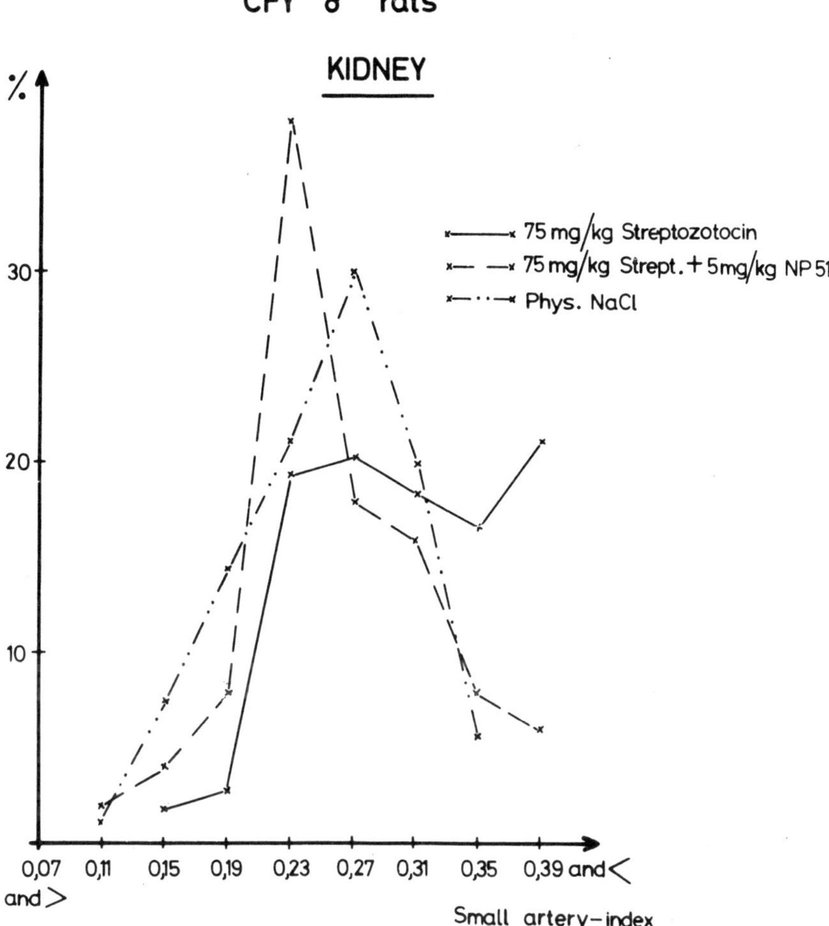

Fig. 3. Vascular-indices of renal arteries.
Other signs see fig. 1.

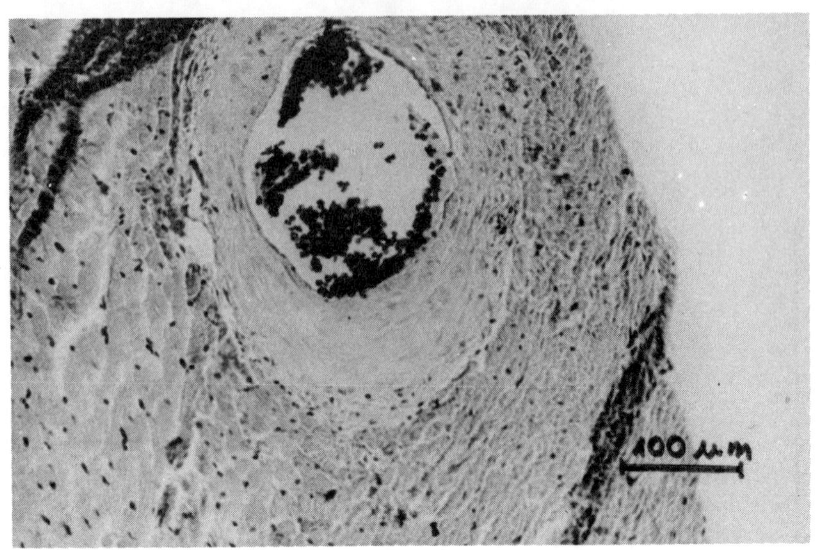

Fig. 4.   Diabetic coronary vessel. Haemalaun-eosin staining.

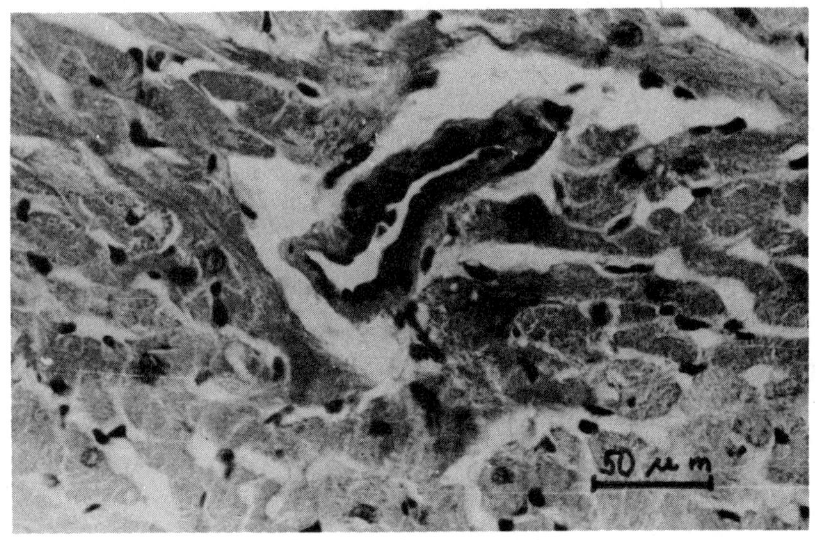

Fig. 5.   Diabetic coronary vessel, pretreated by NP51.
Haemalaun-eosin staining.

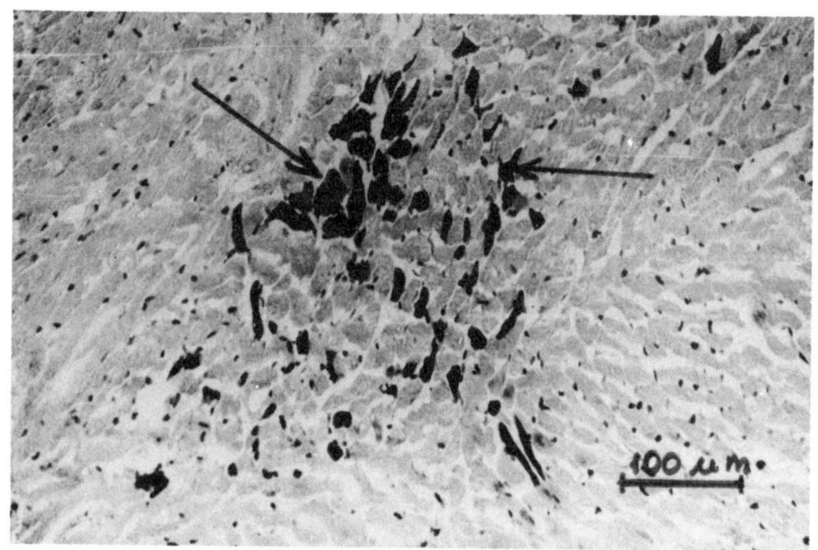

Fig. 6.   Hypoxic myocardium in experimental diabetes.Staining
see methods. Hypoxic areas are dark-spotted.

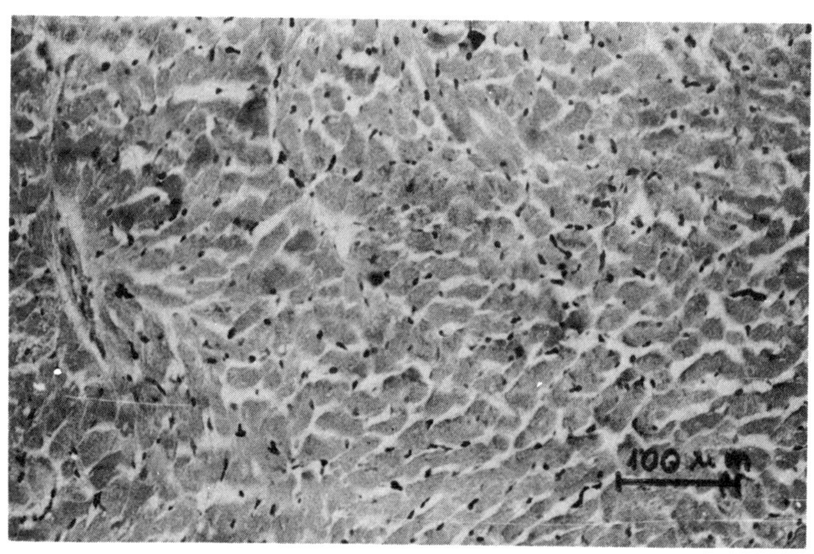

Fig. 7.   Hypoxic staining in a diabetic rat's myocardium
pretreated by NP51.

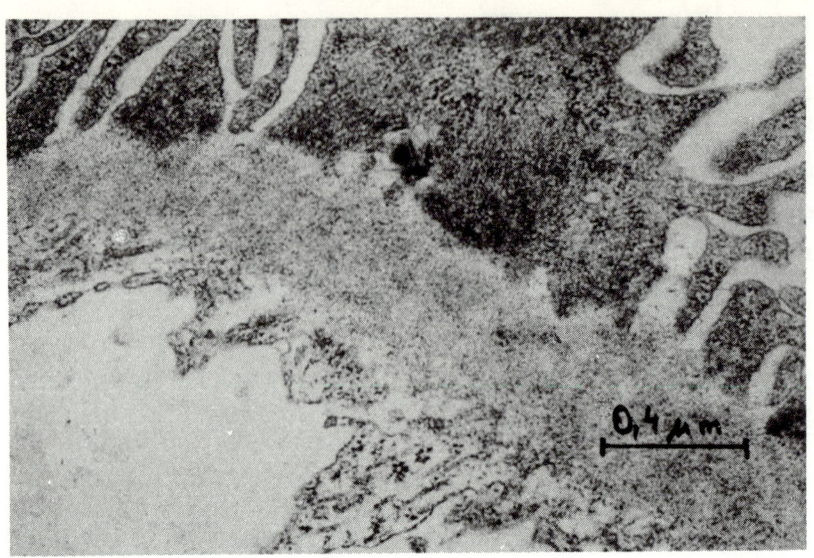

Fig.8. Electronmicrogram. The thickening of the basal
membrane of a glomerulus is seen.

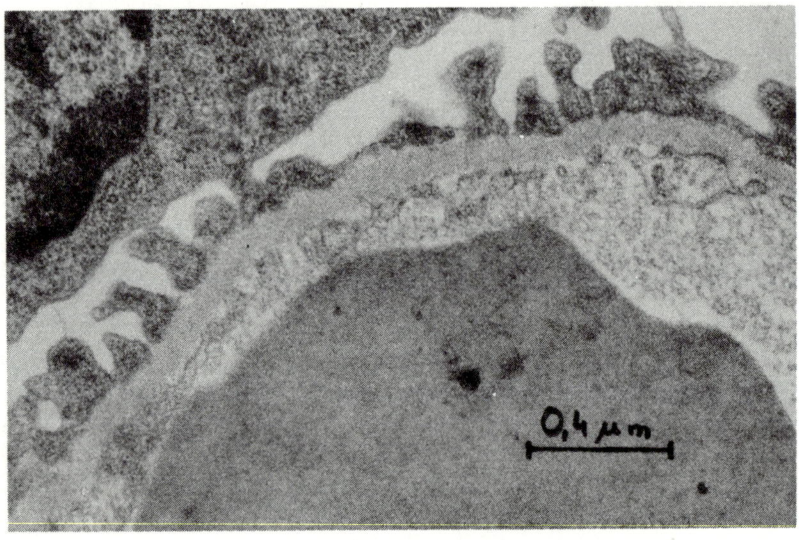

Fig.9. Electronmicrogram of diabetic rat's glomerular
basal membrane. The animal was treated with NP51.

210

<u>Pogátsa</u>: How can a chemical substance bring about changes in morphological events?

<u>Vértesi</u>: First of all the development of morphological changes can be prevented. If the pathological substances are freshly deposited they can be removed.

ALTERED ADRENERGIC RESPONSE
OF THE CORONARY AND FEMORAL ARTERIAL
BED IN ALLOXAN-DIABETIC DOGS

G. Pogátsa
Research Unit, National Institute of Cardiology, Budapest, Hungary

Diabetes mellitus is known to cause disturbed blood flow pattern in the coronary and peripheral arteries and a number of well-characterized morphological changes in the heart and in the limbs /Bentley et al., 1973; Goethals et al., 1975; Gunderson, 1974; McMillan, 1975; Stricht et al., 1974; Tingaud et al., 1974/. The vascular deterioration and altered blood flow patterns may be caused directly by diabetes-induced metabolic defects. Another possibility is that these processes are mediated by early changes in vascular smooth muscle reactivity to vasoactive neurotransmitters or circulating hormones. In this respect, Brody and Dixon /1964/ found increased constrictor responses to catecholamines, but not to sympathetic stimulation in the hindquarters of the diabetic rat. However, Christlieb /1974/ found normal norepinephrine pressor sensitivity in diabetic rats. The same group /Christlieb et al., 1976/ later reported slightly decreased norepinephrine sensitivity in uncomplicated human diabetics, but somewhat increased responsiveness to the catecholamine after the development of diabetic retinopathy. A recent study found increased catecholamine-induced release of vasodilator prostaglandin-like substances in isolated diabetic rat hearts /Stam and Hulsman, 1977/. In the present study, therefore, dogs with alloxan-diabetes were examined for adrenergic response in the coronary and femoral arterial vascular bed.

MATERIALS AND METHODS

Healthy mongrel dogs of both sexes, weighing 16-18 kg, 2-3
years of age, were selected for the study. The dogs were dewor-
med and they had no clinical evidence of disease in four weeks
of observation before the study began. Blood samples were negative for heart worms and both hematocrit and serum albumin were
initially normal. All dogs received the same diet consisting of
15% fat, 25% protein and 60% carbohydrate.

At the beginning of the experiment urine samples collected over
24 hours were tested for glucose /Hyvärinen and Nikkilä, 1962/
and acetone /Neuweiler, 1933/. Fasting venous blood samples were
also taken for determination of glucose /Hyvärinen and Nikkilä,
1962/ and urea nitrogen /Coulombe and Favreau, 1963/. The plasma disappearance rate of glucose /Conard et al., 1953/ was determined by intravenous challenge of 1 g/kg glucose in the unanesthetized state. After determination of the basal values
twelve dogs were made diabetic without ketosis using alloxan
tetrahydrate /Merck/ 60 mg/kg intravenously, given sequentially
for two doses at two weeks intervals. Twelve dogs served as
controls. During the experiment, body weight and 24-hour urinary glucose and acetone excretion were measured at least once
weekly, and the chemical variables of fasting venous blood were
determined at least once monthly.

The hemodynamic investigation was performed 3-month after the
induction of diabetes. One day before the hemodynamic investigation, all chemical variables and the plasma disappearance rate of glucose were redetermined again, than in six control and
in six alloxan-diabetic animals the anterior descending branch
of the left coronary artery and in other six control and in
other six alloxan-diabetic dogs the left femoral artery was exposed under pentobarbital anesthesia /Nembutal, Serva, 30 mg/kg
intravenously/ and the blood flow of the respective artery was
measured by an electromagnetic flowmeter /Type SP 2202, Godard-
-Statham/. Arterial blood pressure was determined in the right
femoral artery. For drug administration the respective artery
was cannulated 10 mm distally from the place of blood flow mea-

surement by Seldinger technique in the case of femoral artery
or through a collateral branch in the case of coronary artery
with a polyethylene venous catheter /Type No 13210, Vygon/. After determination of the basal values, at first norepinephrine
/l-norepinephrine bitartrate, Burroughs Wellcome/ then isoprenaline /l-isoprenaline hydrochloryde, Cilag-Chemie/ and finally
epinephrine /l-epinephrine tartrate, Burroughs Wellcome/ was
perfused into the artery in 2.5-5.0-10.0-20.0 ng/kg/min doses
by a peristaltic pump /Type 5098, MTA KUTESZ/. Each dose of catecholamine perfused as long as equilibration period developed,
usually in five minutes. Subsequently 1 μg/kg/min isoprenaline
was infused intravenously for 30 minutes in order to long-last-
ing stimulation of the beta-adrenergic receptors. After the re-
turning of the initial values of the hemodynamic variables the
dose-response curves of norepinephrine and isoprenaline were
redetermined again.

Paraffin sections of the femoral and coronary arterial wall, of
the myocardium and of the gastrocnemius muscle were used for
histological study, after fixation in formaline or Carnoy fixa-
tive. The sections were stained for PAS-reaction, with Gömöri's
silver stain, and a part of these was exposed to digestion by
diastase. Frozen sections were stained for lipids with Sudan
III or Sudan black.

The results were evaluated statistically using Student's paired and unpaired t-test and regression analysis.

RESULTS

The fasting blood glucose level of the dogs rose durably and
considerably /$p < 0.001$/, while the computed value of the plasma disappearance rate of glucose decreased significantly
/$p < 0.01$/ under the influence of treatment with 2x60 mg/kg alloxan. Urinary glucose excretion rose to a corresponding degree, but acetone was not excreted. Body weight decreased by
about 12% /$p < 0.05$/ following alloxan treatment. These data demonstrated that a clinically manifest diabetes developed without ketosis /Fig. 1/.

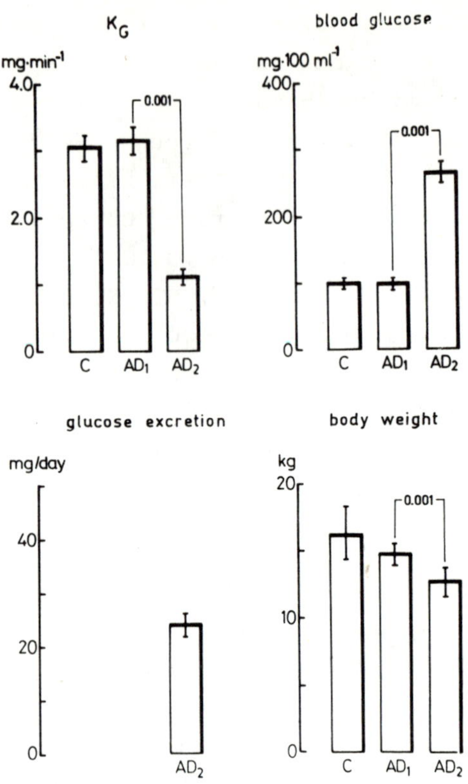

Fig. 1. Effect of alloxan on metabolic variables. Each value is the mean + S.E.M. of twelve animals. K_G = plasma disappearance rate of glucose; C = values of control animals just before hemodynamic investigation; AD_1 = = values of animals before alloxan treatment; AD_2 = values of alloxan-diabetic animals before hemodynamic investigation.

Arterial blood pressure decreased significantly /$p < 0.01$/ both in the control and in the alloxan-diabetic animals, while the blood flow of femoral artery increased in the control group only during the intravenous infusion of 30 µg/kg isoprenaline. After infusion the arterial blood pressure increased /$p < 0.001$/ and the blood flow of the femoral artery decreased /$p < 0.05$/ in both groups /Fig. 2/.

During the coronary artery investigations a similar alteration was found in the blood pressure under the influence of 30 µg/kg isoprenaline, but the coronary blood flow increased not only

216

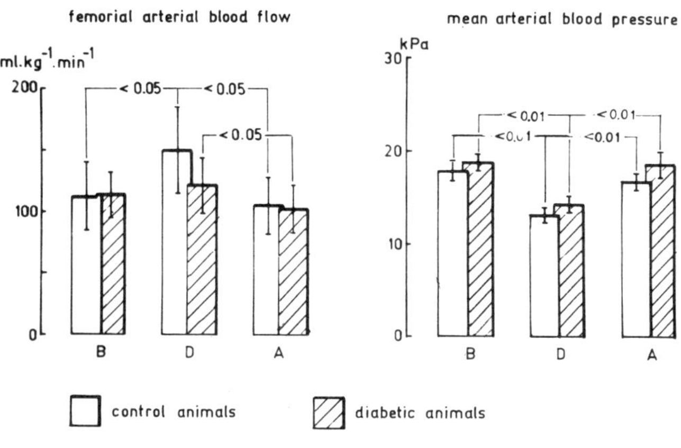

Fig. 2. Effect of intravenous isoprenaline infusion on femoral arterial blood flow and blood pressure. Each value is the mean $\pm$ S.E.M. of six animals. B = values before the intravenous isoprenaline infusion; D = values during the intravenous isoprenaline infusion; A = values after the intravenous isoprenaline infusion.

in the control, but in the diabetic animals, too. After intravenous infusion the increase of blood pressure and the decrease of blood flow were in both groups similar to the alterations of femoral investigations /Fig. 3/.

The dose-response curves of isoprenaline-induced alterations in the vascular conductance of the femoral arterial bed were similar in the control and in the alloxan-diabetic groups before the intravenous isoprenaline infusion. Whereas, after the intravenous isoprenaline infusion the slope became more steeper in the control animals and somewhat flatter in the alloxan-diabetic dogs. Accordingly, a significant /p < 0.01/ difference developed under the influence of 30 µg/kg isoprenaline between the control and the alloxan-diabetic animals in the slopes of isoprenaline-induced dose-response curves. In contrast to this phenomenon, the slope of norepinephrine-induced dose-response curve was somewhat /p = 0.05/ steeper in the alloxan-diabetic group than in the control animals before the intravenous isoprenaline infusion. However, this difference disappeared under

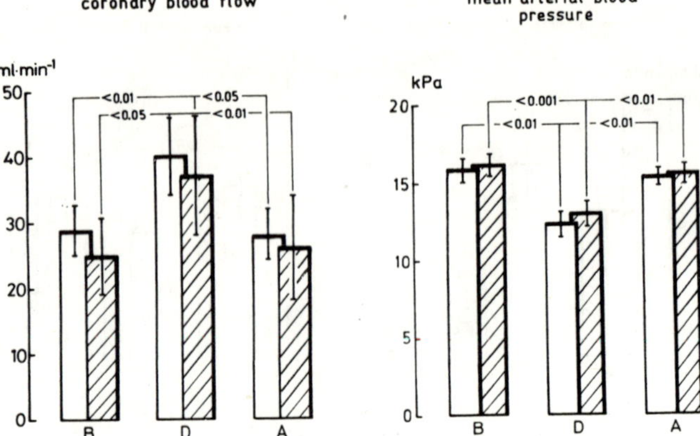

Fig. 3. Effect of intravenous isoprenaline infusion on coronary blood flow and blood pressure. Each value is the mean ± S.E.M. of six animals. B = values before the intravenous isoprenaline infusion; D = values during the intravenous isoprenaline infusion; A = values after the intravenous infusion.

the influence of 30 µg/kg isoprenaline because the slope of norepinephrine-induced dose-response curve became steeper in the control group, too /Fig. 4/.

In the case of coronary artery the slopes of the dose-response curves of isoprenaline-induced alterations in the vascular conductance were somewhat steeper in the control dogs than in the alloxan-diabetic animals before the intravenous isoprenaline infusion. Under the influence of 30 µg/kg isoprenaline, however, the difference between the slopes became somewhat greater between the two gruops. Furthermore, in the case of coronary arteries the slope of the dose-response curves of norepineph-rine-induced alterations in the vascular conductance was essen-tially different before intravenous isoprenaline infusion. That is to say, that the slope of control animals tended to upwards, while the slope of alloxan-diabetic animals tended to downwards. This fact documented that norepinephrine produ-ced a definite vasodilatation in the coronary arteries of con-

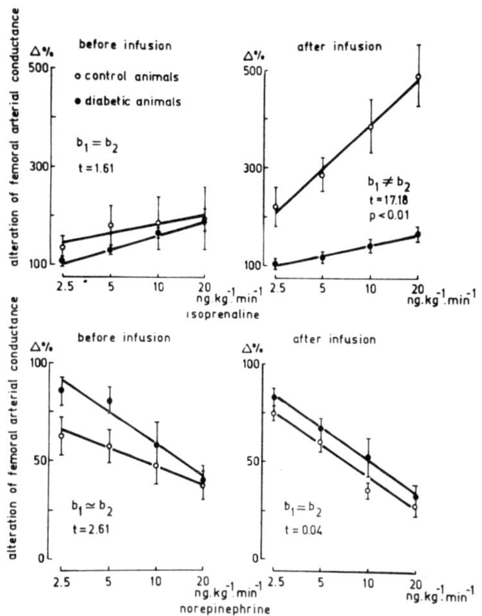

Fig. 4. Dose-response curves of isoprenaline- and norepinephrine-induced alterations in the vascular conductance of the femoral arterial bed. Each value i s the mean $\pm$ S.E.M. of six independent experiments. b = numerical value of the slope of the linear regression /y = a + bx/.

trol animals and a definite vasoconstriction in alloxan-diabetic dogs. After intravenous isoprenaline infusion the difference disappeared because the slope of the control dogs turned down, too /Fig. 5/.

The dose-response curves of epinephrine-induced alterations in the vascular conductance of coronary arteries were in every respect similar to those of isoprenaline-induced alterations /Fig. 6/.

Histologically neither the femoral nor the coronary arterial

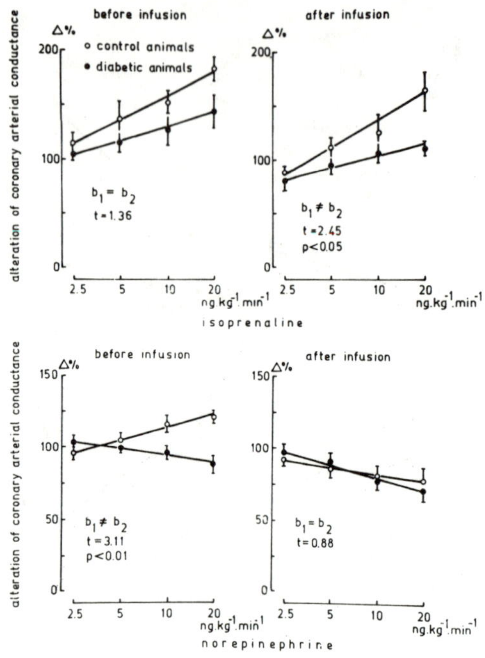

Fig. 5. Dose-response curves of isoprenaline and norepinephrine-induced alterations in the vascular conductance of the coronary arterial bed. Each value is the mean $\pm$ S.E.M. of six independent experiments. b = numerical value of the slope of the linear regression /y = a + bx/.

wall, the gastrocnemius muscle or the myocardium showed any abnormality. The capillary wall and the basement membranes of capillary vessels and muscle fibers were not hypertrophic, and lipid-like materials had not accumulated in the tissues.

DISCUSSION

Our present observations demonstrated that in diabetic condition a tendency to reduced vasodilatation is detectable in the coronary and femoral arterial bed . This phenomenon could be produced by several causes.

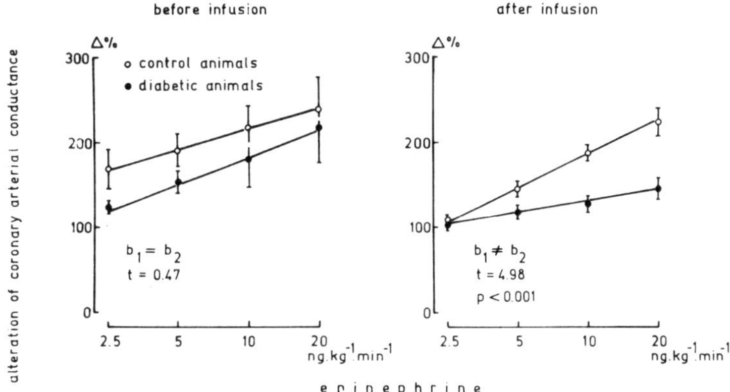

Fig. 6. Dose-response curves of epinephrine-induced alterations in the vascular conductance of the coronary arterial bed. Each value is the mean ± S.E.M. of six independent experiments. b = numerical value of the slope of the linear regression /y = a + bx/.

A possible explanation is that atherosclerotic or microangiopathic alterations of the arterial wall are responsible for the reduced vascular conductance of the diabetic arterial bed. This possibility was precluded in our investigation by the histological examinations.

Another possible explanation is that the beta adrenergic receptor activation is reduced in the vessel wall of diabetic beings. This possible alteration could also be produced by several causes. The cause of the reduced diabetic receptor activation to isoprenaline could be, for example, the decreased concentration of catecholamines in the vicinity of the adrenergic receptors of the diabetic smooth muscle cell, leading to decreased beta receptor activation. Another possible cause could be a decreased affinity of diabetic beta adrenergic receptors for catecholamines. A further possible cause could be that the mechanism of reduced diabetic responsiveness is somewhere in the chain of events starting at the beta adrenergic receptors and ending with the contractile proteins. However, Sullivan and Sparks /1979/ could not support these hypotheses in the aortic strips of diabetic rabbits.

Another possible explanation is that diabetes results in reduced substrate availability, causing decreased ATP production. This interpretation is suggested by the findings that glycolysis is the major energy production pathway and alloxan-diabetes causes significantly decreased glucose uptake and decreased lactate production /Mulcahy and Winegrad, 1962/.

A further remaining explanation is that vasodilatation in the diabetic arterial wall is limited by a change in contractile protein function. This possibility is supported, on one hand, by the observation that protein synthesis is merkedly reduced in the muscle of alloxan-diabetic animals /Newsholme and Start, 1973/. On the other hand, previous observations found in diabetes mellitus a definitely increased stiffness in the arterial wall /Huston and Abboud, 1962; Pillsbury et al., 1974/, in the skin /Caulfield, 1972/, in the lungs /Schuyler et al., 1976/ and in the heart /Pogátsa et al., 1979/. This phenomenon includes contribution from both contractile and elastic elements to passive components in these tissues. Accordingly, a possible explanation of the decreased vasodilatation of the diabetic arteries may be associated also with this fact.

Finally, the interconversion theory /Kunos and Szentiványi, 1968; Kunos, 1977/ may be a further explanation of the reduced vasodilatation of diabetic arteries. Kunos /1977/ demonstrated, namely, a significant shift from alpha to beta adrenergic receptor function in hyperthyreotic rat myocardium, while Preksaitis and Kunos /1979/ disclosed an inverse shift in the regulation of liver glycogen phosphorylase enzyme. Because of the preliminary nature of our approach, experiments on the static and dynamic mechanical properties of diabetic vessels are in progress. These studies might reveal changes in adrenergic receptor, smooth muscle or vessel wall mechanics that could explain the reduced responsiveness of diabetic arterial bed to isoprenaline.

SUMMARY

Dose-response curves of norepinephrine- and isoprenaline-induced alterations in the vascular conductance of the coronary and femoral arterial bed have been investigated in twelve clinically manifest, but nonketotic, alloxan-induced diabetic dogs and in twelve healthy control animals, before and after intravenous infusion of 1 μg/kg/min isoprenaline for 30 minutes. Alloxan, 2x60 mg/kg, was administered intravenously 3 month before the hemodynamic investigations were performed. Intravenous infusion of 30 μg/kg isoprenaline enhanced the effect of intraarterially administered isoprenaline on vascular conductance of the coronary and femoral arterial bed in the control animals only, while in diabetic dogs it was ineffective. The effect of intraarterially administered norepinephrine was different on the vascular conductance of the coronary arterial bed in the control and alloxan-diabetic animals. Before intravenous isoprenaline infusion, norepinephrine produced a definite vasodilatation in the coronary arteries of control animals, and a definite vasoconstriction in the alloxan-diabetic animals. After intravenous isoprenaline infusion the difference disappeared because norepinephrine produced vasoconstriction in the control dogs, too. Vascular atherosclerosis, microangiopathy could be ruled out on the basis of histopathological examination.

REFERENCES

Bentley,P.J., Candia,O.A., Parisi,M., Saladino,A.J. /1973/ Effects of hypoormolality on transmural sodium transport in the toad bladder. Amer.J.Physiol. <u>225</u>: 818-824.

Brody,M.J., Dixon,R.L. /1964/ Vascular reactivity in experimental diabetes mellitus. Circ.Res. <u>14</u>: 494-501.

Caufield,J.B. /1972/ Dermal elastic tissue of diabetics. Beitr.Pathol. <u>145</u>: 286-296.

Christlieb, A.R. /1974/ Renin, angiotensin, and norepinephrine in alloxan diabetes. Diabetes <u>23</u>: 962-970.

Christlieb,A.R., Janka,H., Kraus,B., Gleason,R.E., Icasas-Cabral,E.A., Aieilo,L.M., Cabral,B.V., Solano,A. /1976/ Vascular reactivity to angiotensin II and to norepinephrine in diabetic subjects. Diabetes 25: 268-274.

Conard,V., Franckson,J.R.M., Bastenie,P.A., Kestens,J., Kovács, L. /1953/ Étude critique du triangle d'hyperglycémie intraveineux chez l'homme normal et détermination d'un coefficient d'assimilation glucidique. Arch.Int.Pharmacodyn. 93: 277-292.

Coulombe,J.J., Favreau,L. /1963/ A new simple semimicro method for colorimetric determination of urea. Clin.Chem. 9: 102-108.

Goethals, M.A., Adele,S.M., Brutsaert, D.L. /1975/ Proceedings: Osmolality and myocardial function. Arch.Int.Physiol.Biochim. 82: 756-758.

Gunderson,H.J. /1974/ Peripheral blood flow and metabolic control in juvenile diabetes. Diabetologia 10: 225-231.

Huston,J.H., Abboud,F.M. /1962/ Measurement of arterial aging in relation to diabetes mellitus. Circulation 25: 938-946.

Hyvärinen,A., Nikkilä,E.A. /1962/ Specific determination of blood glucose with o-toluidine. Clin.Chim.Acta 7: 140-143.

Kunos,G. /1977/ Thyroid hormone-dependent interconversion of myocardial alpha- and beta-adrenoreceptors in the rat. Brit. J.Pharmacol. 59: 177-189.

Kunos,G., Szentiványi,M. /1968/ Evidence favouring the existence of a single adrenergic receptor. Nature 217: 1077-1078.

McMillan,D.E. /1975/ Deterioration of the microcirculation in diabetes. Diabetes 24: 944-953.

Mulcahy,P.D., Winegrad,A.I. /1962/ Effects of insulin and alloxan diabetes on glucose metabolism in rabbit aortic tissue. Am.J.Physiol. 203: 1038-1042.

Neuweiler,W. /1933/ Quantitative Bestimmung der Acetonkörper im Blut mittels des Stufenphotometers. Klin.Wschr. 12: 869-980.

Newsholme,E.A., Start,C. /1973/ Regulation in Metabolism, edited by E.A. Newsholme and C. Start, 1st ed. Wiley, London, p. 129, 330-331.

Pillsbury,H.C., Hung,W., Kyle,M.C., Freis,E.D. /1974/ Arterial

pulse waves and velocity and systolic time intervals in diabetic children. Amer.Heart J. __87__: 783-790.

Pogátsa,G., Bihari-Varga,M., Szinay,Gy. /1979/ Effect of diabetes therapy on the myocardium in experimental diabetes.
Acta Diabetol.Lat. __16__: 129-138.

Preiksaitis,H.G., Kunos,G. /1979/ Adrenoceptor - mediated activation of liver glycogen phosphorylase: effects of thyroid
state. Life Sci. __24__: 35-42.

Schuyler,M.R., Niewoehner,D.E., Inkley,S.E., Kohn,R. /1976/
Abnormal lung elasticy in juvenile diabetes mellitus. Amer.
Rev.Respir.Dis. __113__: 37-41.

Stam,H., Hulsman,W.C. /1977/ Effect of fasting and streptozo-
tocin-diabetes on the coronary flow in isolated rat hearts:
a possible role of endogenous catecholamines and prostaglandins /Abstract/. Basic,Res.Cardiol. __72__: 365-375.

Stricht,van der J., Ledant,P., Vanhove,J. /1974/ Diabetic arte-
riopathy - nosolic entity. J.Cardiovasc.Surg. __15__: 62-67.

Sullivan,S., Sparks,H.V. /1979/ Diminished contractile response
of aortas from diabetic rabbits. Amer.J.Physiol. __236__: H301-
H306.

Tingaud,R., Masse,C.L., Boissieras,P., Baste,J.C., Plagnol,Ph.
/1974/ Diabetic ateriopathies. J.Cardiovasc.Surg. __15__: 54-61.

DISCUSSION

Szentiványi: I think Dr Pogátsa's work confirms and extends
our former results concerning the pathophysiologic transformation of beta-adrenoceptor effects in diabetes. This transformation apparently diminishes the propensity of vessels for
vasodilation, and, in doing so, forms the functional basis of
diabetic angiopathy.

Pogátsa: I agree. The vessels of our animals did not manifest
even the preliminary signs of morphologic changes which are
characteristic of advanced forms of diabetes. Interesting e-
nough even at this stage the beta-vasodilator system does not
function normally.

Kunos: Your results show a beautiful example of thorough pharmacologic analysis of hind limb adrenoceptors in experimental
diabetes. Have you any further evidence for the reciprocal behaviour of alpha and beta effects?

Pogátsa: If I interpret your question aright you are suggesting evidence for interconversion of adrenoceptors according
to the theory of yours. As I stressed formerly in my paper,
every aspect of our results are perfectly compatible with your
one-receptor theory, although they do not prove it directly.

Juhász-Nagy: In sharp contradistinction with the beta-adrenoceptors of the femoral arterial bed, coronary receptors of the
normal dogs did not show the signs of an increased sensitivity
to beta-agonists after infusion of isoproterenol in massive
doses /compare right upper panels of your Fig. 4. and 5./. This
probably means an increased sensitivity to tachyphylaxis of
coronary beta-effects, as it was found in our experiments, too
/see Papp et al., this symposium/.

Pogátsa: I think your interpretation is correct. Since the
alpha/beta adrenergic balance in the coronaries swings to the
beta-side more than in the circulation of resting skeletal
muscle, tachyphylaxic-resistant reserves of adrenoceptors in
the latter territory should be more pronounced than in the
former one. However, I cannot document this surmise, it is
simply a hypotesis.

SOME ASPECTS OF MYOCARDIAL NORADRENALINE METABOLISM IN THE ISCHEMIC RAT HEART

I. Préda, M. Sebeszta and Z. Antalóczy
2nd Medical Clinic and Central Research Laboratory, Postgraduate Medical School, Budapest, Hungary

Numerous clinical and experimental observations have shown an increased sympathetico-adrenal activity during the early stage of myocardial infarction (Harris et al., 1951; Staszewska-Barczak and Ceremuzynsky 1968; Jewitt et al., 1969). Blood catecholamine concentration is significantly increased on the first two days following coronary occlusion and is accompanied by increased catecholamine excretion (Valori et al., 1967; Nelson, 1970; Lukomsky and Oganov, 1972). Similarly, it was shown that catecholamine concentration is already elevated in the first 10 minutes after coronary ligation in dogs (Richardson, 1963), and the noradrenaline (NA) level in the effluent of the coronary sinus is higher after coronary ligation (Kárpáti and Préda, 1973).

A high concentration of catecholamines in the normal heart was recorded by a number of investigators (Potter and Axelrod, 1963; Iversen, 1963; von Euler and Lishajko, 1965) and the NA content was found to exceed that of adrenaline and dopamine (Angelakos et al., 1969). Regional distribution of catecholamine content in the atria and the ventricular muscle as well as its localisation in the neuronal and non-neuronal elements in widely discussed in the literature (Michaelson et al., 1964; Snyder et al., 1964; Hamberger, 1965; Bensome and Berger, 1971).

It is also known, that 17-spironolactones, which are potent inhibitors of aldosterone have some direct effects on the isolated mammalian myocardium, such as a positive inotropic effect on cat papillary muscle (Tanz and Kerby, 1961), a lengthening of the functional refractory period, an antifibrillatory effect and a decrease in transmembrane efflux of potassium in rabbit atria (Briggs and Holland, 1959), and a lengthening of the intracellular action potential of guines pig atria (Bacciarelli, 1967). Coraboeuf and Deroubaix (1974) reported on a similar direct action on the isolated heart tissue of sodium cancrenoate, structurally related to spironolactones but with no lactone ring. Furthermore potassium cancrenoate causes a reversal of oubain-induced electrophysiological effects in isolated Purkinje fibers (Yeh and Lazarra, 1973), and increases stroke volume and left ventricular output in the coronary ligated canine heart (Kötter et al., 1975).

In the present investigations we have studied the uptake of labelled NA by the heart muscle following coronary occlusion in rats and the influence of potessium-cancrenoate (Aldactone) on the uptake and metabolism on the normal and hypopotassemic rat myocardium.

Methods

A total of 312 R Amsterdam male rats of 180 to 240 g was used in the study.

Coronary occlusion was performed in ether anaesthesia according to the technique of Selye. The whole surgical procedure was performed within approximately 60 seconds. In sham-operated animals thoracotomy was performed, the pericardium was incised with a fine scissors and the heart was exteriorized. More than 80% of the operated rats survived the coronary ligation.

The animals were killed by decapitation in the 10th, 30th and 60th minutes, and 4 and 14 days after coronary ligation.

^{14}C-NA (methylene-^{14}C-dl-noradrenaline bitartrate, 47 μCi/mM, Amersham) was injected in a quantity of 0,7 μCi/100 g in 0,1 ml physiological saline solution into the tail vein at the time of, or, in other groups, in the 60th minute after coronary ligation. The animals were sacrificed in the 10th, 30th and 60th minute after NA treatment.

In further groups, the uptake of labelled NA was studied on the 4th
and 14th postoperative days when the animals were killed 1 hour after
the NA injection. In all cases the blood pH determination from systemic blood was made by the micro-Astrup method.

After careful washing in physiological saline the left ventricle
was divided into ischemic, peri-ischemic and visibly intact zones,
about 20 mg specimens were excised and placed in 2,5 ml ethanol-0,1
M HCl solution (4:1). After homogenization in a glass homogenizer the
samples were centrifuged and the supernatant evaporated in counting
vials. Radioactivity was measured in 10 ml Bray solution with a
Packard 340 EX liquid-scintillation spectrometer.

In the studies in vitro, 50 mg specimens from the left ventricle
were placed in 2,0 ml Tyrode's solution containing 0,1% ascorbic acid
as antioxydant. The incubation medium was adjusted to pH 6,8 and 7,1
by 0,05 M acetic acid. After administration of 0,005 and/or 0,01 μCi
labelled NA the specimens were incubated in a shaker at 37 $^{\circ}$C for
30 minutes. Then the tissue pieces were carefully washed in an excess
of the incubation medium without labelled NA. The uptake of radio-
active NA was measured as described above.

For studying the effect of potassium-cancrenoate (Aldactone,
Boehringer) on NA uptake and NA content of the rat heart, the animals
were anaesthetised with pentobarbital, then were given 5 mg/100 g
spironolactone intraperitoneally 10 and 30 minutes before NA determination. The control animals equal volumens of physiological saline were
given.

Intracellular potassium loss was induced by daily intraperitoneal
administration of 1 mg/100 g furosemide during a 3-week period.

Fluorometric assay of myocardial NA content was done by the
method of <u>Udenfried</u> and <u>Zaltman-Nierenberg</u> (1963).

For studying ^{3}H-NA (10,6 μCi/mmol, Amersham) uptake, 0,5 -
1,5 μCi/100 g labelled NA was diluted in 0,2 ml physiological saline
and injected into the tail vein of the anaesthetised rats. Thirty minutes
later they were killed by decapitation, the atrial and ventricular tissues

were dissected out, and from about 30 mg pieces of the tissues the extraction of NA was carried out according to the above mentioned method.

In certain experimental series, monoamino-oxydase activity was blocked by mg/100 g pargyline given 30 minutes prior to the injection of ^{3}H-NA.

Intracellular potassium was estimated by flame photometry after wet ashing by HNO_3 hydrogen proxide; usually 20-30 mg myocardial tissue was ashed for parallel determinations.

For statistical evaluation of the data the Student's t test was applied.

<u>Results</u>

A marked increase of labelled NA uptake was observed after coronary ligation. Total uptake of the non-ischemic zones in the 10th, 30th and 60th minutes showed a decline following coronary occlusion, but the activity was still significantly higher than in the sham-operated rats (Fig. 1.). In the coronary ligated rats the blood pH reached its normal range in the 30th minute.

The distribution of radioactivity in the ischemic, peri-ischemic and non-ischemic zones of the left ventricle showed significant differences in the rats killed in the 10th minute after coronary occlusion. The macroscopically intact tissue had accumulated much more NA than did the ischemic or peri-ischemic zones (Fig. 2.).

NA uptake was then estimated at 2 hours, 4 days and 14 days following coronary ligation. In the ischemic and peri-ischemic zones the level fell below the initial value on the 14th day (Fig. 3.), and in the macroscopically intact zone to the initial value.

For studying the possible role of acidosis in the events, normal heart tissue specimens were incubated at different pH levels. In competition studies, the administered excess amount of unlabelled NA (10^{-7} M per incubation medium) was replaced by labelled NA approximately to the same extent at pH 6,8 and pH 7,4 (Fig. 4.). In further experiments, significantly more NA was accumulated at pH 6,8

230

than at pH 7,4 but there was no statistically significant difference between the values at pH 7,1 and pH 7,4 (Fig. 5.).

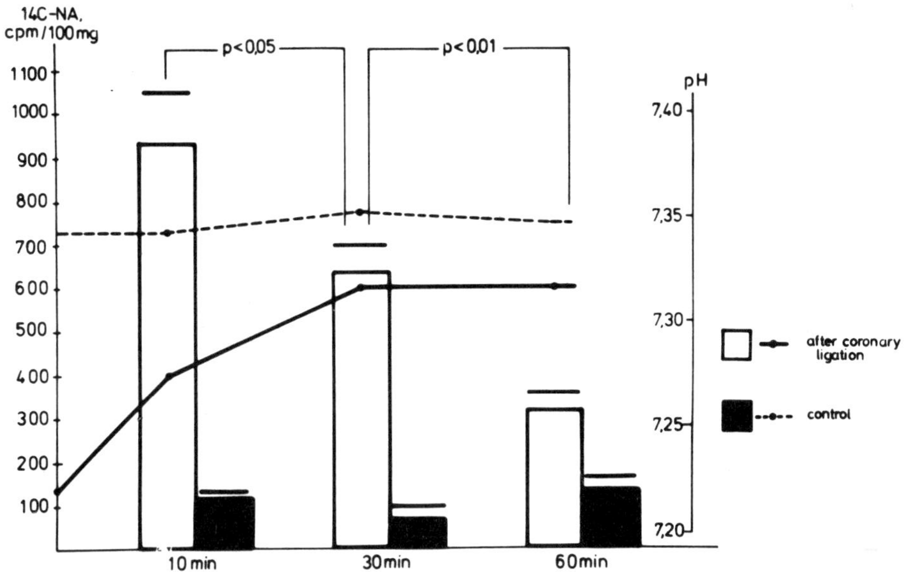

Fig. 1. NA concentration is non-ischemic myocardial tissue after coronary ligation in rats. The values obtained in sham-operated animals were used as controls

Spironolactone administered 30 minutes before the injection of labelléd NA caused a marked increase of the radioactive catecholamine pool in both the ventricular and atrial tissues (Fig. 6.).

Pargyline pretreatment augmented the effect of spironolactone on ^{3}H-NA uptake in the ventricular tissue. Pargyline alone caused a significant rise in the accumulation of radioactive catecholamine in the ventricular tissue (Fig. 7).

Fluorometric determination showed no significant differences in ventricular NA content between spironolactone pretreated and untreated groups (Fig. 8.).

A higher NA uptake with an unchanged NA content suggested an increased rate of NA turnover as a result of spironolactone treatment.

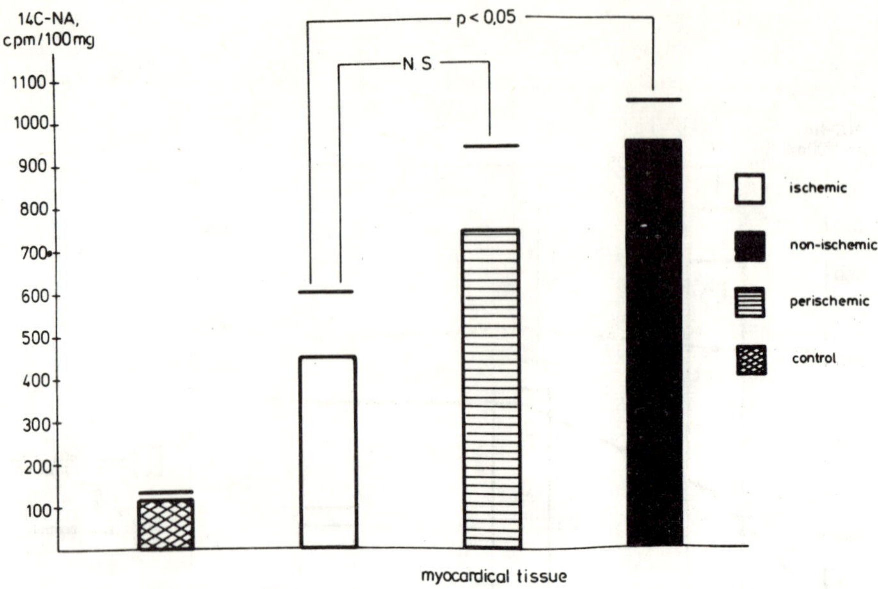

Fig. 2. Regional differences in the accumulation of labelled nor-adrenaline after coronary ligation; the values have been compared to those of shame-operated controls. The animals were killed 10 minutes after coronary ligation.

For studying the possible role of a low intracellular potassium level on the mechanism of the spironolactone effect, rats were treated with furosemide for 3 weeks. There was a significant decrease in the potassium content of the ventricular tissue (56,3 - 37,8 mEq/kg). Spironolactone administration 60 minutes before decapitation resulted in a restoration of the intracellular potassium (37,8 - 59,8 mEq/kg) concentration (Fig. 9.).

^{3}H-NA uptake by the ventricular tissue was significantly less after furosemide treatment. Spironolactone administration 30 minutes prior to the tracer injection led to the normalization of the catecholamine pool.

Spironolactone pretreatment 10 minutes before the injection of labelled NA led to a similar but slighter increase in the uptake (Fig. 10.).

232

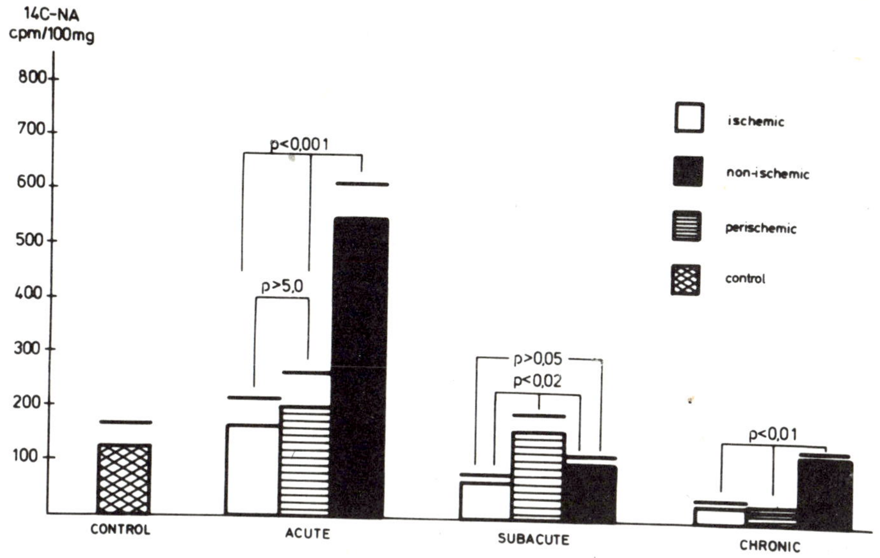

Fig. 3. Accumulation of labelled NA in different zones of the myocardium after coronary ligation. The values were obtained at 120 minutes, 4 and 14 days after coronary ligations. In the acute period, labelled noradrenaline was given in the 60th minute after ligation.

Discussion

NA is considered the predominating catecholamine compound of the mammalian heart; its higher concentration in the atria than in the ventricle in explained by the denser sympathetic nervous supply of the atrial tissue (Angelakos et al., 1969) NA exerts a positive influence on coronary blood flow, muscular contractility and the pacemaker function of the sinus node. In pathological conditions or in high doses, its negative effect on the heart performance cannot be neglected.

Preliminary studies on rats suggested that the myocardial NA concentration was markedly increased in metabolic acidosis (Kárpáti et al., 1975). Moreover, in metabolic acidosis induced by coronary ligation an increased uptake of circulating catecholamines was observed

(Préda _et al._, 1975).

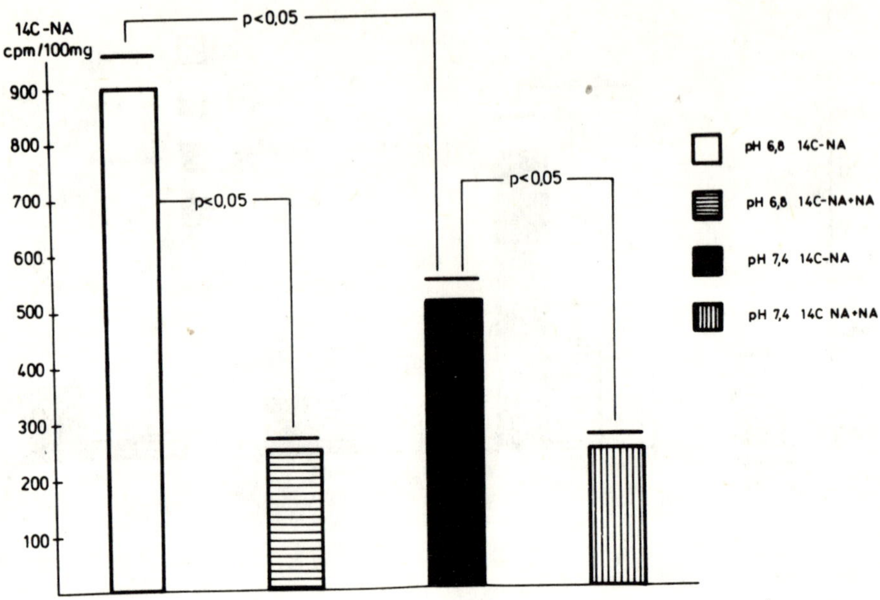

Fig. 4. Competition of unlabelled NA with accumulation of radio-active NA at different pH levels. Labelled NA uptake was supressed by the addition of 10^{-7} M NA to the incubation medium.

In the present study, myocardial NA accumulation was significantly more marked in the coronary ligated than is sham-operated animals. The increased uptake cannot be attributed solely to the effect of extracellular acidosis as a temporary consequence of coronary ligation, as the phenomenon may be observed in the subacute period, too. Moreover, a transient intracellular acidosis as a causative factor in the increased NA uptake by both the intact and the ischemic zones may also be taken into consideration.

According to our experimental results, spironolactone significantly increased NA turnover in the myocardium, as suggested by an increased uptake and an unchanged NA content of the heart.

An increased NA turnover due to the effect of spironolactone may explain the positive inotropic property as well as the antifibrillatory effect of the ccmpound. NA is well known to have a role in the activation of cAMP as a second messenger of the positive inotropic effect of catecholamines (Sutherland et al., 1968).

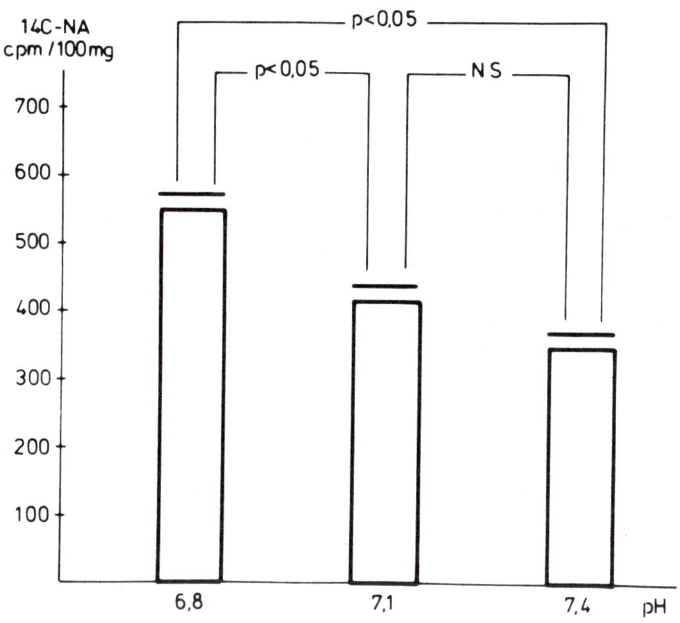

Fig. 5. NA uptake by myocardial tissue at different pH levels.

Concerning the mechanism of the catecholamine effect, an influence on the ionic currents across the cardiac cell membrane was assumed (Reuter, 1967; Vassort et al., 1969). A current flow through the "fast" (tetradotoxin-sensetive) sodium channel responsible for the initial rapid phase of depolarization is not modified appreciably by adrenaline, although it increases significantly the slow inward Na^+ and Ca^{++} current which can be blocked by manganese ions (Hagiwara and Nakijama, 1966; Coraboeuf and Vassort, 1968). This effect seems to be responsible for the development of the plateau of the action potential and also for the appearence of action potential overshoot. The latter effect may account for the observation that adrenaline increases the plateau amplitude of the action potential recorded from different heart regions (Carmeliet and Vereecke, 1969) as reflected by an augmented relative refractory period. This ought to be taken into account in the mechanism of the antifibrillatory effect of catecholamines under certain circumstances.

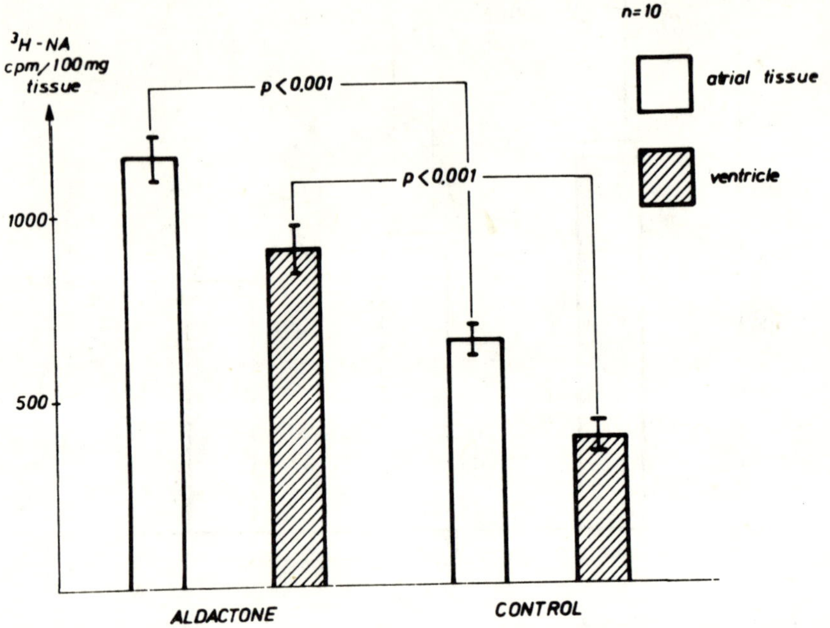

Fig. 6. Effect of 5 mg/100 g spironolactone on ^{3}H-NA uptake by atrial and ventricular tissues. Spironolactone was administered intraperitoneally 30 minutes before the radioactivity determination procedure.

As <u>Iversen</u> (1965) has shown, two different processes are involved in the accumulation of catecholamines: $uptake_1$ and $uptake_2$. $Uptake_1$ is related mainly to a catecholamine accumulation in neuronal alaments, while $uptake_2$ is linked mainly to non-neuronal tissues. The blockade of non-neuronal catecholamine uptake ($uptake_2$) was demonstrated by the administration of different steroids such as desoxycorticosterone (Salt, 1972). The present observations led to assume that the increased NA uptake induced by spironolactone is due to its antialdosterone property and is mediated through an augmented non-neuro-nal (uptake$_2$) process while an unchanged endogenous catecholamine pool would indicate a greater participation of uptake$_1$.

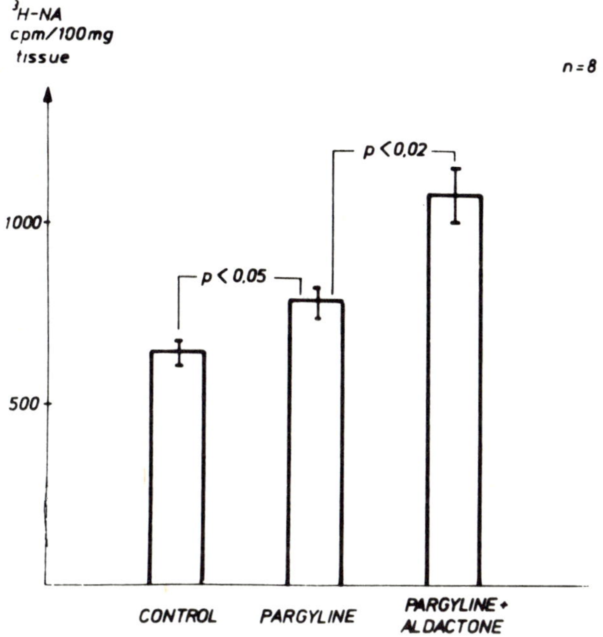

Fig. 7. Pargyline pretreatment by prevention of NA degradation causes a marked increase in ^{3}H-NA uptake of ventricular tissue as compared to the controls.

According to the present results, an increased NA uptake and turnover rate may play a role in the positive inotropic and antiarrhythmic effect of spironolactone. We suggest that its positive inotropic property is mediated by an increased NA uptake and turnover rate while the antiarrhythmic effect might be explained by its influence on ionic currents, as reflected by an augmentation of the relative refractory period. The latter effect is improved by restoration of the intracellular potassium level in saluretic treated rats.

The role of catecholamines in the maintenance of pump function is well known. The elevation of the blood catecholamine level as well as the increased NA accumulation in the heart muscle after coronary

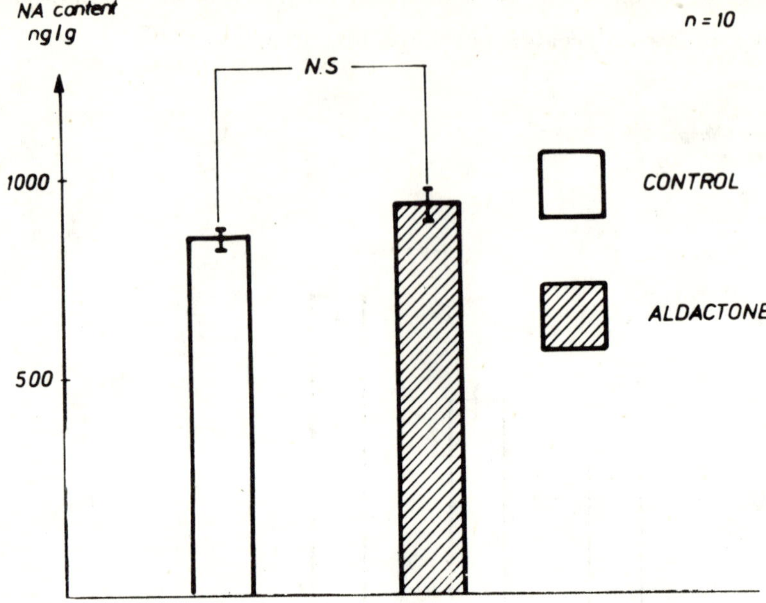

Fig. 8. Fluorometrically determined NA content of ventricular tissue on normal and spironolactone pretreated rats (N.S.: non significant)

occlusion must not be interpreted exclusively as a positive effect on heart function. There are numerous observations to show that the catecholamines at physiological concentrations exert a positive influence on coronary blood flow, muscular contractility and pacemaker function although beyond a certain limit their negative effect on the heart cannot be excluded. Arrhythmia can be prevented by beta blocking agents (Hayasky and Penney, 1969; Khan et al., 1972). These observations also raised the possibility of a negative influence of an increased catecholamine supply on heart function in myocardial damage.

<u>Summary</u>

Coronary ligation produced a marked increase in labelled noradrenaline uptake in the myocardial tissue of rats. The periischemic zones showed an elevated accumulation of noradrenaline on the 4th day

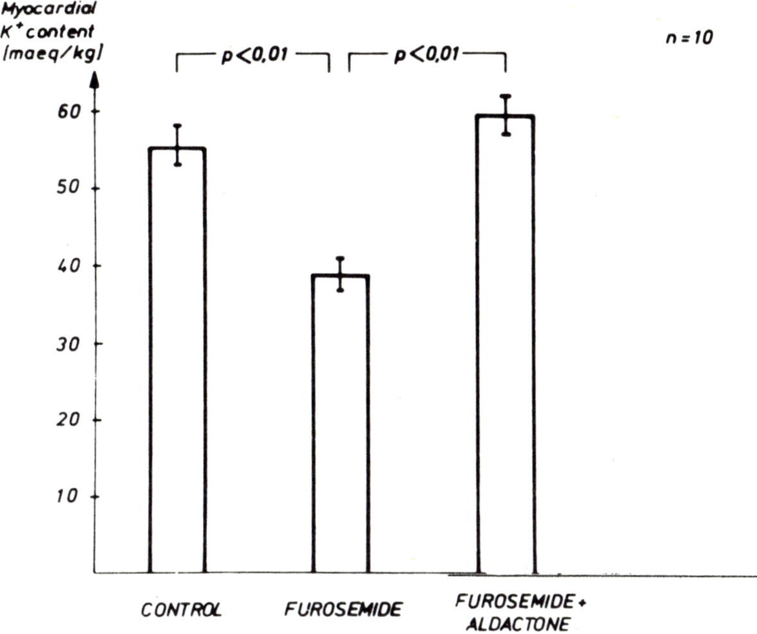

Fig. 9. Furosemide pretreatment induced a significant loss in intracellular potassium content of the ventricular tissue. Spironolactone administration 30 minutes before the assay has normalized the intracellular potassium content.

when the intact zone had returned to normal values. At the 14th day of observation, both the ischemic and peri-ischemic tissue exhibited a subnormal accumulation of radioactivity. Intracellular acidosis was probably involved in the enhanced accumulation of noradrenaline in the damaged myocardium. In further studies the influence of potassium-canrenoate on the noradrenaline uptake and metabolism were studied in normal and hypopotassemic rats. In normal rats spironolactone administration resulted in a marked increase of labelled noradrenaline uptake, but the noradrenaline content remained unchanged. In saluretic-pretreated animals spironolactone normalized both the previously decreased noradrenaline uptake and low intracellular potassium level of the heart tissue. The augmentation of catecholamine metabolism due to spironolactone may be involved in enhanced activity of adenyl cyclase and forms the basis of the positive inotropic effect of the compound.

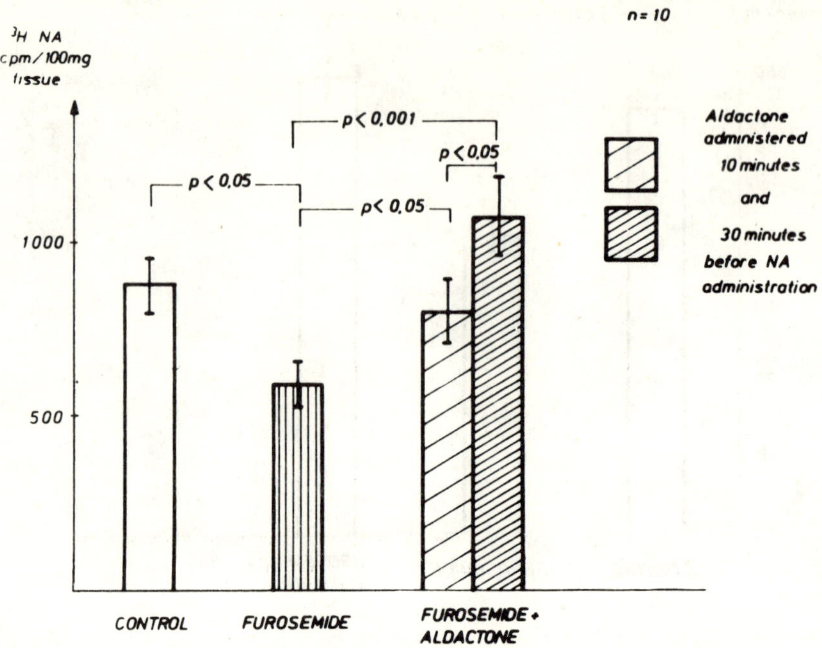

Fig. 10. 5 mg/100 g spironolactone administered 10 and 30
minutes before the NA uptake assay. There is an increase in
^{3}H-NA uptake of the ventricular myocardium, which is more
marked in animals receiving spironolactone 30 minutes before
the study.

References

Allen, J.D., Pantridge, J.F., Shanks, R.G.: Practolol in the treatment of ventricular dysrhythmias in acute myocardial infarction.
Postgrad. Med. J., 1971. Suppl. 47: 29-31.

Angelakos, E. T., King, M. P., Millard, R. W.: Regional distribution of catecholamines in the hearts of various species. Ann. N.Y.
Acad. Sci., 1969. 156: 219-240.

Bensome, S. A., Berger, J. M.: Specific granules in mammalian and
non-mammalian verebrate cardiocytes. In: Bajusz, E., Jasmin, G.
(Eds): Methods and Achievements in Experimental Patology. Karger,
Basel 1971, Vol. 5. pp. 173-213.

Bacciarelli, C.: L'effetto della digoxina, del dessossicorticosterone e dello spironolactone sul miocardio di mammifere. Arch. int. Pharmacodyn. _166:_ 150-166 (1967).

Briggs, A. H., Holland, W. C.: Antifibrillatory effects of electrolyte regulating steroids on isolated rabbit atria. Amer. J. Physiol. _197:_ 1161-1164 (1959).

Carmeliet, E., Vereecke, J.: Adrenaline and the plateau phase of the cardiac action potential. Pflügers Arch. ges. Physiol. _313:_ 300-315 (1969).

Coraboeuf, E., Vassort, G.: Effect of some inhibitors of ionic permeabilities on ventricular action potential of rat and guinea-pig hearts. J. Electrocardiol. _1:_ 19-30, 1968.

Coraboeuf, E., Deroubaix, E.: Effect of spironolactone derivative, sodium cancrenoate, on mechanical and electrical activities of isolated rat myocardium. J. Pharmacol. exp. Ther. _191:_ 128-138, 1974.

von Euler, E. S., Lishajko, F.: Free and bound noradrenaline in the rabbit heart. Nature (Lond.) _105:_ 179-180, 1965.

Farnebo, L. O., Malmforms, T.: Histochemical studies on the uptake of noradrenaline and alpha-methylnoradrenaline in the perfused rat heart. Europ. J. Pharmacol. _5:_ 313-320, 1969.

Hagiwara, S., Nakijama, S.: Differences in Na and Ca spikes as examined by application of the tetradotoxine, procaine and manganese ions. J. gen. Physiol. _49:_ 793-806, 1966.

Hamberger, B.: Reserpine resistant uptake of catecholamines in isolated tissues of the rat. A histochemical study. Acta physiol. scand. suppl. _295:_ 1-64, 1965.

Harris, A. S., Estandia, A., Tillotson, R. F.: Ventricular ectopic rhytms and ventricular fibrillation following cardiac ympathectomy and coronary occlusion. Amer. J. Physiol. _165:_ 505-512, 1951.

Hayasky, K. D., Penney, D. P.: Catecholamine metabolism in early myocardial infarction. Circulation suppl. _40:_ 103, 1969.

Iversen, L. L.: The uptake of noradrenaline by the isolated perfused rat heart. Brit. J. Pharmacol. _21:_ 523-537, 1963.

Iversen, L. L.: The uptake of catecholamines at high perfusion concentrations in the isolated rat heart; a novel catechclamine uptake process. Brit. J. Pharmacol. _25:_ 18-33, 1965.

Jewitt, D. E., Mercer, C. J., Ried, D., Valori, C., Thomas, M., Shillingford, F. P.: Free noradrenaline and adrenaline excreation in relation to the development of cardiac arrhythmias and heart failure in patients with acute myocardial infarction. Lancet, <u>1</u>: 635-641, 1969.

Kárpáti, P., Préda, I.: Experimentális szivizom-anyagcsere vizsgálatok coronaria ligatura után. Cardiol. Hung. <u>2</u>: 137-146, 1973.

Kárpáti, P., Préda, I., Endrőczi, E.: Effect of acidosis and noradrenaline infusion on ^{14}C-noradrenaline uptake by the rat myocardium. Acta physiol. Acad. Sci. Hung. <u>46</u>: 99-106, 1975.

Khan, M., Hamilton, J. T., Manning, G. W.: Protective effect of beta adrenoreceptor blockade in experimental coronary occlusion in consicious dogs. Amer. J. Cardiol. <u>30</u>: 832-837, 1972.

Kötter, V., Leitner, E. v., Arbeiter, G., Cordes, R., Schröder,R.: Der Einfluss von Cancrenoat-Kalium (Aldactone pro injectione) auf Haemodynamik und Myokardischaemie beim experimentellen Myokardinfarkt. Z. Kardiol. <u>64</u>: 672-686, 1975.

Lukomsky, P. E., Oganov, R. G.: Blood plasma catecholamines and their urinary excretion in patients with acute myocardial infarction. Amer. Heart J. <u>83</u>: 182-188, 1972.

Michaelson, I. A., Richardson, K. C., Snyder, S. N., Titus, E. O.: The separation of catecholamine storage vesicles from rat heart. Life Sci. <u>3</u>: 971-978, 1964.

Nelson, P. G.: Effect of heparin on serum free fatty acids, plasma catecholamines and the incidence of arrhythmias following acute myocardial infarction. Brit. med. J. <u>3</u>: 735-737, 1970.

Potter, L. T., Axelrod, J.: Properties of norepinephrine storage particles of the rat heart. J. Pharmacol. exp. Ther. <u>142</u>: 299-305, 1963.

Préda, I., Kárpáti, P. Endrőczi, E.: Myocardial noradrenaline uptake after coronary occlusion in the rat. Acta Physiol. Acad. Sci. Hung. <u>46</u>: 99-106, 1975.

Reuter, H.: The dependence of slow inward current in Purkinje fibers on the extracellular calcium concentrations. J. Physiol. (Lond.) <u>192</u>: 492-497, 1967.

Richardson, J. A.: Plasma catecholamine concentrations in acute infarction. In: Lihoff, W., Moyer, J. H. (Eds): Coronary Heart Disease. Grune and Stratton, New York, pp. 273-277, 1963.

Salt, P. J.: Inhibition of noradrenaline Uptake$_2$ in the isolated rat heart by steroids, Clonidine and methoxylated phenethylamines. Europ. J. Pharmacol. <u>20</u>: 329-340, 1972.

Snyder, S. H., Michaelson, I. A., Musacchio, J.: Purification of norepinephrine storage granules from rat heart. Life Sci. <u>3</u>: 965-970, 1964.

Staszewska-Barczak, J., Ceremuzynsky, L.: The continuous estimation of catecholamine release in the early stages of myocardial infarction. Clin. Sci. <u>34</u>: 531-539, 1968.

Sutherland, E. W., Robinson, A. G., Butcher, R. W.: Some aspects of the biological role of adenosine 3', 5'-monophosphate (Cyclic AMP). Circulation <u>37</u>: 279-305, 1968.

Tanz, R. D., Kerby, C. F.: The inotropic action of certain steroids upon isolated cardiac tissue; with comments on steroidal cardiotonic structure activity relationships. J. Pharmacol. exp. Ther. <u>131</u>: 56-64, 1961.

Udenfried, S., Zaltman-Nierenberg, P.: Norepinephrine and 2,4-dihidroxyphenylethylamine turnover in guinea-pig brain in vivo. Science <u>142</u>: 394-396, 1963.

Vassort, G., Roupier, O., Garnier, D., Sauviat, M. P.; Coraboeuf, E., Gargouil, Y. M.: Effect of adrenaline on membrane inward currents during the cardiac action potential. Pflügers Arch. ges. Physiol. <u>309</u>: 70-81, 1969.

Valori, C., Thomas, M., Shillingford, J. P.: Free noradrenaline and adrenaline excreation in relation to clinical syndromes following myocardial infarction. Amer. J. Cardiol. <u>20</u>: 605-617, 1967.

Yeh, B. K., Lazzara, R.: Reversal of ouabain-induced electrophysiological effects by potassium cancrenoate in canine Purkinje fibers. Circulat. Res. <u>32</u>: 501-508, 1973.

ALPHA-ADRENOCEPTORS IN ISCHEMIC CANINE HEART BLOCKED BY PHENTOLAMINE

D. M. Aviado and A. Juhász-Nagy

*Department of Pharmacology, University of Pennsylvania Medical School, Philadelphia, Penn., USA
and National Institute of Vascular Surgery, Semmelweis University Medical School, Budapest, Hungary*

In the mammalian heart, both alpha and beta adrenoceptors are known to exist; both elicit an increase of ventricular contractility, whereas beta adrenoceptors dilate and alpha constrict the coronary blood vessels. Under ordinary circumstances the prevalent effect of adrenoceptor stimulation reflects beta stimulation. The experimental demonstration of the existence of alpha adrenoceptors in the mammalian myocardium and coronary bed has been made chiefly on animal preparations which had their beta receptors blocked with propranolol or other similar drugs.

This is a report of another way of demonstrating alpha adrenoceptor activity without employing beta blocking agents. We have used myocardial ischemia for altering the adrenoceptor quality in a circumscribed venticular region of the in situ canine heart. The nature of the effects have been shown to be altered by changes in myocardial metabolism. An increase in metabolism caused a predominance of beta receptors, a decrease in predominance of alpha receptros in the myocardium (Kunos and Szentiványi, 1968) and in the coronary blood vessels (Szentiványi et al., 1970a; Juhász-Nagy et al., 1974; Juhász-Nagy and Kudász, 1975). The present experiments show that the occlusion of a major coronary branch for a prolonged period of time induces a predominance of alpha adrenoceptors which reflects the low metabolic rate of the damaged myocardial cells.

Methods

General Procedure

Mongrel dogs weighing 11 to 24 kg were anesthetized with intravenous pentobarbital sodium (30 mg/kg). A tracheal canula was inserted and the lungs were ventilated with a positive pressure respirator (Starling Ideal pump) using room air. The heart was approached through a left thoracotomy performed in the fourth intercostal space. The pericardium was slit anterior to the left phrenic nerve from its base to the diaphragm to expose the myocardium. Blood pressure was measured in the ascending aorta through a polyethylene catheter introduced via the left common carotid artery. In order to measure left ventricular pressure, another polyethylene catheter was inserted into the left ventricular cavity through the apex. Both pressures were measured with P23 AA Statham transducers. Mean arterial pressure was obtained by electrical integration. Maximum rate of rise of left venticular pressure (dp/dt max) was displayed using a derivative computer (8814AHP). The recordings were made on a six-channel Sanborn 7700 recorder.

A short segment of the left anterior descending coronary artery, close to its origin, was carefully dissected free. Special precautions were taken to keep to a minimum the number of nerve fibers that might be damaged in the vicinity of the vessel. A snare was placed around the coronary artery for subsequent occlusion; the occlusion was accomplished by pulling this thread against the flanged end of a short polyethylene tube. In those experiments (v. i.) where the coronary vascular reactions within the left ventricle were studied a Statham electromagnetic flow probe of appropriate diameter (usually 2 mm) was fitted around the artery proximal to the occluder. The probe was connected to a Statham SP2202 electromagnetic flowmeter. The vascular responses in the coronary bed were characterized by mean flow changes and by flow: pressure relationships (calculated vascular conductance) determined in the late diastolic phase of the cardiac cycle.

In those experiments where the segmental inotropic responses of the myocardium were studied the changes of local contractility were followed by recording the output of small Walton-Brodie strain gauge arches of 120 ohm resistance sewn to the free wall of the left ventricle. Usually two gauges were used. One of them was sutured to the lateral surface of the left ventricular base supplied by the circumflex coronary artery. The other gauge was placed on the anterior surface close to the apical area, which, according to the distribution of the epicardial branches, was expected to be rendered ischemic by the occlusion of the left anterior descending coronary artery. In some cases, a third gauge was also applied to the right ventricular surface.

Adrenergic activation was effected either by intravenous administration of epinephrine hydrochloride (Adrenalin[R]) or by nerve stimulation. In the latter case, the left stellate ganglion was carefully dissected free, and stimulation of the ansa subclavia was performed with bipolar platinum electrodes. Stimulation was carried out supramaximally (20/sec. 3 msec, 8 to 10 V for stimulation periods 30 to 45 sec) using a Grass S8 stimulator and a Grass stimulus isolation unit. The sensitivity of the myocardium to non-adrenergic inotropic stimuli was tested with intravenous administration of $CaCl_2$ (0. 06 mM/kg).

In order to produce alpha adrenoceptor blockade, phentolamine mesylate (Regitine[R]) was employed in a single dose of 0, 5 mg/kg body weight. The drug was administered by slow i. v. injection over a period of 3 to 4 min duration. The results were examined statistically using

Student's t-test for paired data. All values quoted in the tables and indicated on figures are mean ± standard error.

Experimental Protocol

Two series of experiments were conducted: (1) Determination of the role of the alpha component in the adrenergic inotropic **responses** of ischemic myocardial segments. (2) Characterization of the alpha adrenergic sensitivity in the coronary vascular bed after prolonged occlusion (exposure to ischemia). The specific alpha-blocking capacity of phentolamine was utilized to achieve both ends.

Ischemic heart. In the first series (18 dogs) the left anterior descending coronary branch was occluded at least 1 hour prior to the testing. This procedure diminished considerably the level of local contractility in most cases; the actual experimental measurements started only after a steady state value in the local inotropism had been reached. Coronary occlusion resulted in ventricular fibrillation in 3 out of 21 animals. Survivors, however, exhibited little decrease in arterial blood pressure. In 11 dogs, a dose-response relationship was obtained for epinephrine (0,2; 0,4; and 0,8 μg/kg i.v.), whereas in 10 dogs, the effects of sympathetic nerve stimulation was studied. (Three animals out of 18 were used for both pharmacologic and nervous adrenergic activation as well; in 8 dogs only the pharmacologic and in 7 dogs only the nerve stimulation was investigated.) The respective type of adrenergic stimulus was repeated in every case after alpha blockade with phentolamine.

Post-ischemic heart. In the second series of experiments, the adrenergic vascular responses of the left anterior descending coronary branch have been studied immediately after the cessation of the reactive hyperemic flow increase which followed the prolonged arterial occlusion of 60 to 75 min duration. (Usually 5-10 min were required for the hyperemic response to disappear.) The adrenergic responses of the post-ischemic vessels were compared to those of unoccluded coronary arteries in control animals. Successful experiments were performed in a total of 20 dogs (10 controls and 10 ischemic); ventricular fibrillation ensued in two additional animals after releasing the coronary occlusion. The same methods of adrenergic stimulation and alpha adrenergic blockade which were employed in the first series were used in these animals, too. Both pharmacologic and nervous stimuli were utilized in 2 control (out of 10) and in 2 ischemic (out of 10) dogs.

Results

Adrenoceptors of Ischemic Myocardium

The application of two strain gauges allowed a comparison of changes in contractility of two areas; one portion supplied by an artery that was occluded for one hour, and another that was not subjected to ischemia. The ischemic area, supplied by collateral channels, couls still respond to adrenergic stimulation. However, there was a

difference in predominance of alpha adrenoceptors between the ischemic
and nonischemic areas revealed by the administration of phentolamine,
the alpha blocker used in these experiments.

Effects of epinephrine. A pattern of the epinephrine effect in the
control state as well as after alpha adrenergic blockade with phentolamine is shown in figure 1.

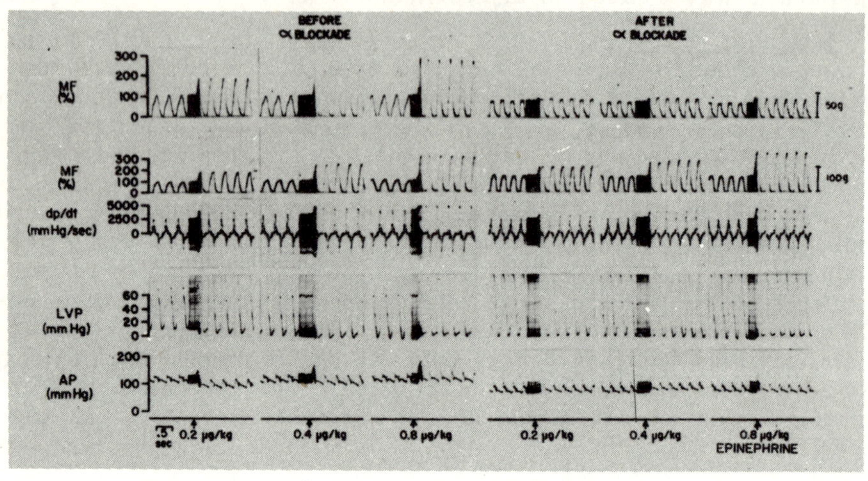

Fig. 1. Effect of alpha-adrenergic blockade with phentolamine
on contractility responses induced by epinephrine. From above
downwards; myocardial contractile force in the ischemic area,
myocardial contractile force in the normal area, dp/dt max,
diastolic portion of the left venticular pressure, arterial blood
pressure.

Before phentolamine administration, both the normal or nonischemic,
and the ischemic regions exhibited comparable magnitude of adrenergic
sensitivity as indicated by the percentage increase of the myocardial
contractile force in the respective area. Alpha blockade proved to be
ineffective in altering the epinephrine response in the normal region.
On the other hand, phentolamine almost completely blocked the inotropic
response to epinephrine in the ischemic portion. This difference revealed after the injection of phentolamine is the basis for the conclusion

248

that ischemic myocardium contains a predominance of alpha receptors, stimulated by epinephrine and blocked by phentolamine; and that the normal or nonischemic myocardium contains a predominance of beta receptors not blocked by phentolamine.

The pattern described above was seen in each of 11 dogs. Figure 2, showing the dose-response curve of the myocardial contractility responses summarizes the results obtained with three doses of epinephrine (0,2, 0,4 and 0,8 µg/kg), before and after alpha adrenoceptor blockade.

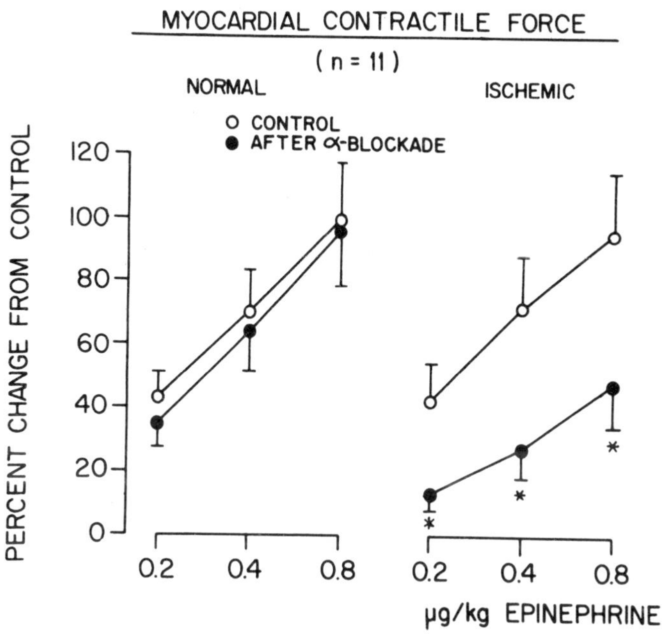

Fig. 2. Dose response relationships of the local inotropic effect of the normal and ischemic myocardial zones before and after alpha-blockade. Mean values ± S. E. Asterisks refer to significance of change after alpha-blockade.

In the normal or nonischemic region, the dose-response relationships remained essentially unchanged after phentolamine (0,5 mg/kg) the slight decrease of adrenergic sensitivity being not statistically significant. In the ischemic myocardial portion, however, alpha-blockade caused the epinephrine dose-response curve to make a shift to the right. The data of table 1 summarizing the behavior of the most important cardiovascular variables of the same experiments, indicate the well-known char-

acteristic features of the epinephrine and phentolamine effects on the
circulation. The data, however, did not reveal any drastic shift in the
level of the basic cardiovascular variables which might have been responsible for the aspecific change of the ischemic contractility responses.

Table 1. Effect of alpha-blockade on circulatory responses induced
          by epinephrine
          (n = 11)

		Control	Change		
Epinephrine dose (μ/kg)			0.2	0.4	0.8
Mean arterial blood pressure (mm Hg)	a	109 ± 4	$+5 \pm 3$	$+13 \pm 3^c$	$+24 \pm 3^c$
	b	82 ± 4^d	-3 ± 1^d	$+2 \pm 1^d$	$+7 \pm 2^{cd}$
Heart rate (beats/min)	a	168 ± 9	$+3 \pm 1^c$	$+7 \pm 1^c$	$+19 \pm 3^c$
	b	190 ± 10^d	$+2 \pm 1$	$+4 \pm 1^{cd}$	$+5 \pm 1^{cd}$
dp/dt max (mm Hg/sec)	a	2052 ± 189	$+1425 \pm 295^c$	$+2359 \pm 409^c$	$+3550 \pm 510^c$
	b	2284 ± 189	$+775 \pm 168^{cd}$	$+1386 \pm 297^{cd}$	$+3550 \pm 404^c$
Myocardial contractile force, normal (g)	a	87 ± 7	$+35 \pm 5^c$	$+58 \pm 9^c$	$+86 \pm 14^c$
	b	86 ± 9	$+30 \pm 7^c$	$+53 \pm 10^c$	$+80 \pm 14^c$
Myocardial contractile force, ischemic (g)	a	54 ± 8	$+18 \pm 4^c$	$+32 \pm 7^c$	$+49 \pm 12^c$
	b	50 ± 8	$+6 \pm 3^{cd}$	$+13 \pm 4^{cd}$	$+21 \pm 7^{cd}$

a Before alpha-blockade
b After alpha-blockade
c Significant change (p < 0.05) from pre-stimulation control
d Significant change (p < 0.05) after alpha-blockade

Effects of sympathetic nervous stimulation. The behavior of contractility responses induced by sympathetic nerve stimulation was found
to be analogous to that of the pharmacologically-induced responses.
Figure 3 shows a typical experiment. Supramaximal stimulation of the
left anterior ansa increased the contractile force both in the normal or
nonischemic, and the ischemic myocardial regions. After the injection
of phentolamine, the response in the normal zone remained unchanged,
while it was blocked in the ischemic zone. In fact, as opposed to the

control contractility response, a decrease in inotropism could be observed in the latter zone after alpha blockade, probably reflecting the distracting forces of the surrounding normal regions.

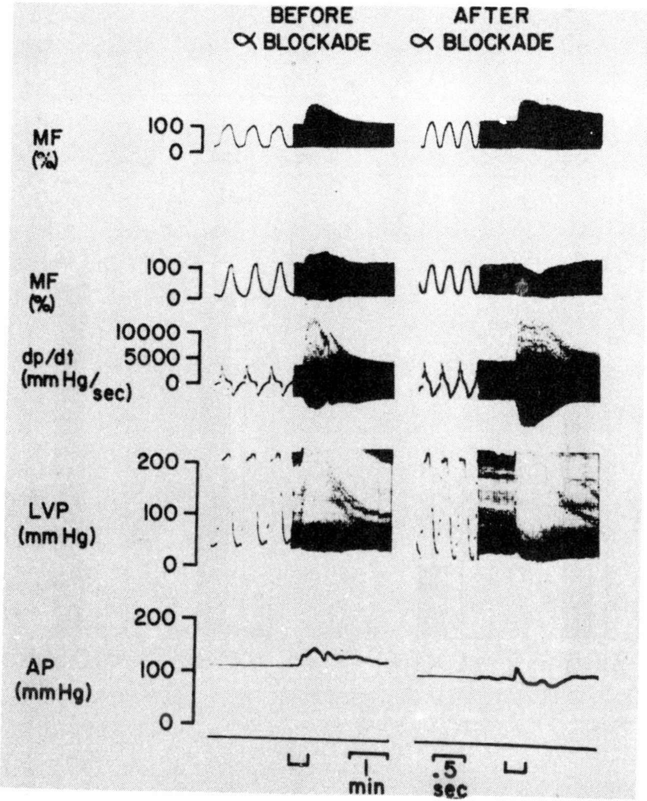

Fig. 3. Effect of alpha-blockade on contractility responses induced by sympathetic stimulation. From above downwards; myocardial contractile force in the normal region, myocardial contractile force in the ischemic region, dp/dt max, diastolic portion of left ventricular pressure, mean arterial blood pressure.

The statistical analysis of a total of 10 similar experiments summarized in figure 4 indicated a significantly modified ischemic contractility response to sympathetic nervous stimulation after alpha-blockade, whereas phentolamine failed to decrease the contractility response of the normal or nonischemic area. Figure 4 also depicts the analysis of inotropic responses to the infravenous injection of calcium chloride (0.06 mM) given to the same animals. The responses remained unchanged after phentolamine in both regions, indicating the specificity of the blockade. The summary of the basic hemodynamic measurements in table 2 also failed to reveal characteristic modifications of the general circulatory equilibrium and its sensitivity to sympathetic nerve stimuli, except the well-known decrease of the mean arterial blood pressure level and a reduced response of heart rate to the stimulus after the injection of phentolamine. The latter change was probably due to an increased basic (pre-stimular) heart rate after alpha-blockade.

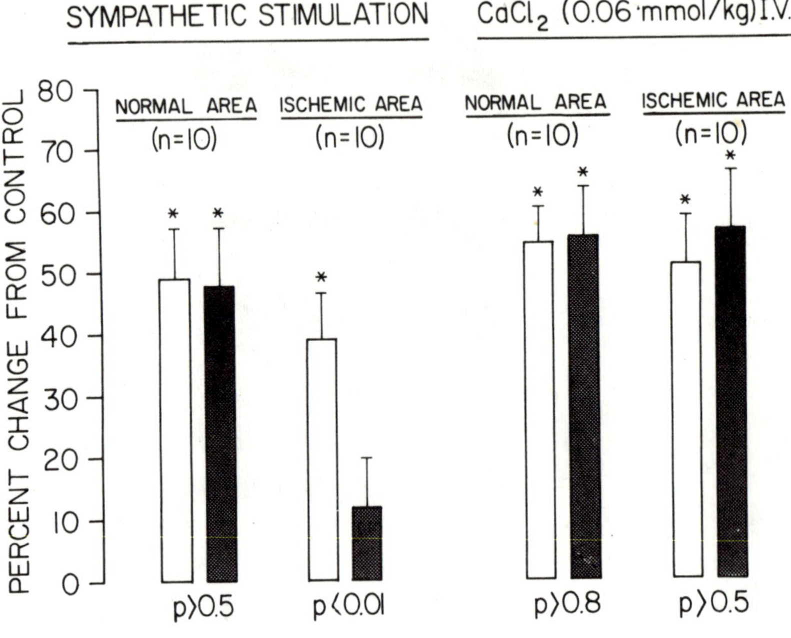

Fig. 4. Comparison of inotropic responses induced by cardiac sympathetic nerve stimulation and Ca^{2+} before (white columns) and after (dark columns) alpha-adrenergic blockade. Mean values $\pm$ S.E. Asterisks refer to the significance of change induced by the stimulus. P-values refer to significance of change induced by alpha-blockade.

Adrenoceptors of the Coronary Blood Vessels

The procedure was modified in the experiments on the coronary circulation to permit measurements of coronary arterial flow. After one hour of arterial occlusion, the ligature was released for the study of coronary blood flow in the post-ischemic myocardium. These post-ischemic adrenergic responses were compared to those of unoccluded anterior descending coronary arteries in control animals.

Effects of epinephrine. Fig. 5. summarizes the results of 6 control experiments performed on normal or nonischemic coronaries, and those of 6 experiments performed in the post-ischemic coronary bed following arterial occlusion of 60 to 75 min duration. In the normal coronary bed, well known diminution of the systemic adrenergic pressor response after alpha blockade by phentolamine is associated with a considerably reduced flow increase; in the post-ischemic bed, this reduction in mean flow response was less obvious, and statistically not significant except for the highest dose administered. In complete accordance with this pattern, after alpha blockade, a significantly enhanced tendency to adrenergic vasodilation could be observed in the post-ischemic coronaries but not in the normal vessels.

Table 2. Effect of alpha-blockade on circulatory responses induced by sympathetic stimulation
(n = 10)

		Control	Change
Mean arterial blood	a	123 ± 5	$+8 \pm 4$
pressure (mm Hg)	b	99 ± 5	-4 ± 2^{d}
Heart rate	a	158 ± 7	$+19 \pm 4^{c}$
(beats/min)	b	181 ± 7	$+ 9 \pm 3^{cd}$
dp/dt max	a	3125 ± 310	$+3375 \pm 708^{c}$
(mm Hg/sec)	b	2950 ± 353	$+3075 \pm 701^{c}$
Myocordial contractile	a	79 ± 8	$+ 40 \pm 9^{c}$
force, normal (g)	b	80 ± 8	$+ 39 \pm 9^{c}$
Myocordial contractile	a	43 ± 3	$+ 17 \pm 3^{c}$
force, ischemic (g)	b	43 ± 5	$+ 5 \pm 4^{d}$

a   Before alpha-blockade
b   After alpha-blockade
c   Significant change ($p < 0.05$) from pre-stiumulation control
d   Significant change ($p < 0.05$) after alpha-blockade

Effects of sympathetic nervous stimulation

We found essentially a similar vascular pattern in adrenergic responses induced by sympathetic nervous stimulation. In the normal coronary bed, supramaximal sympathetic stimulation elicited the usual vasodilator reaction in association with increased cardiac contraction. This coronary vasodilation was consequently but moderately augmented after alpha adrenoceptor blockade by phentolamine. In the post-ischemic coronary circulation, the vasodilator response was less pronounced in the control state but increased considerably after alpha blockade with phentolamine (Fig. 6.).

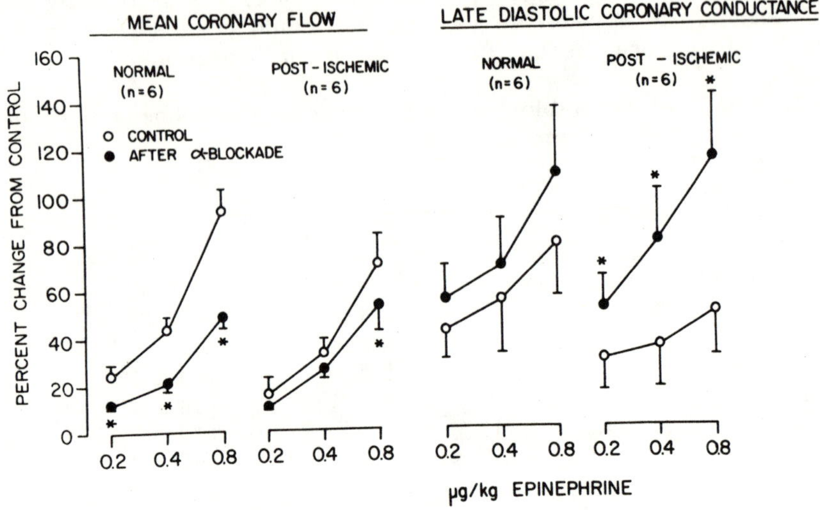

Fig. 5. Dose response characteristics of the epinephrine-effect on the coronaries before and after alpha-blockade. Mean values ± S.E. Asterisks refer to significance of change induced by alpha-blockade.

Discussion

As early as in 1906, Dale recognized that ergot alkaloids were less effective in blocking excitatory cardiac responses produced by epinephrine and nervous stimulation than they were in blocking excitatory (constrictor) responses of the vascular smooth muscle. This original observation has been confirmed and extended by most subsequent investigators; the evidence led Ahlquist (1948) to classify adrenoceptors in the heart as belonging to the beta group. However, from time to time observations were also made indicating that under certain circumstances, alpha adrenoceptor antagonists may be effective against cardiac adrenergic excitation especially in cold-blooded animal species (Amsler, 1920; Nickerson and Nomaguchi, 1950). Although the circumstances underlying the validity of alpha adrenoceptor blockade were not clearly specified, similar potency of alpha antagonists have been reported even against the mammalian adrenergic inotropic responses (Cotten and Walton, 1951 ;

254

Cotten _et al._ , 1957). This striking efficacy of alpha-blocking agents
under certain circumstances have never been explained satisfactorily
by other authors who could not substantiate the observations of Cotten
and her co-workers.(Moran and Perkins, 1961; Nickerson and Chan,
1961; Newman, 1976).

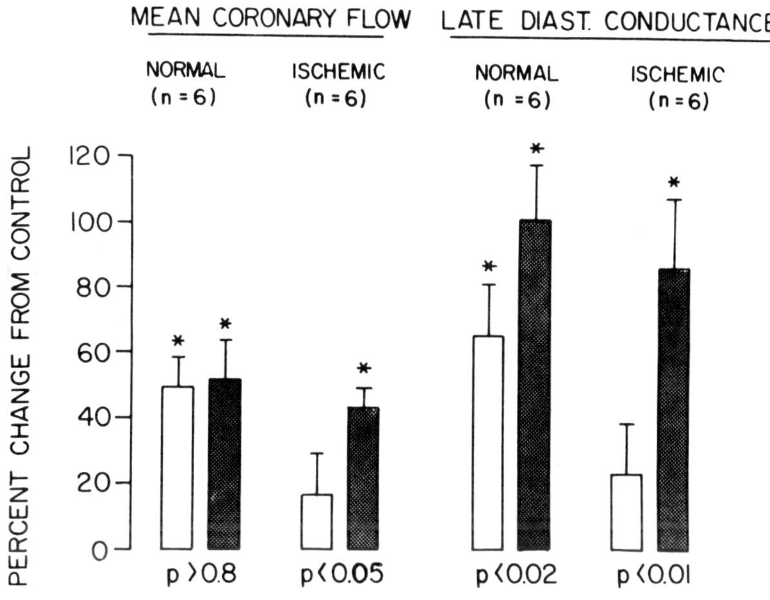

Fig. 6. Effect of alpha-blockade on coronary responses to sympathetic nerve stimulation before (white columns) and after (dark
columns) alpha-adrenoceptor blockade. Mean values ± S.E. Asterisks refer to significance of change induced by the stimulus.
P-values refer to significance of change induced by alpha-blockade.

The discovery of effective and highly specific beta blocking agents in-
augurated a temporary requiescence in the field of this apparent confu-
sion. Subsequently, there were challenges of the widely accepted concept that cardiac adrenoceptors are all beta in nature. It has been con-
clusively demonstrated that an increase of cardiac contractile activity
also can be induced by alpha adrenoceptors. (Govier _et al._ , 1966;
Wenzel and Su, 1966; Govier, 1968; Benfey, 1973; Wagner _et al._ ,
1974). It may rightly be assumed that the relative contribution of alpha
and beta adrenoceptor mechanisms to the overall excitatory adrenergic
response could be modified by several factors.

The present experiments indicate the increased role of the alpha component in the adrenergic effects of the ischemic myocardium. Although our experiments failed to prove any significant difference between the relative sensitivity of the normal and the acutely ischemic canine myocardium to adrenergic stimuli before alpha blockade, a clear distinction has been established in this respect after phentolamine administration. Phentolamine injection reduced the adrenergic contractility increase within the ischemic myocardial area. Therefore, in contrast to the normal or nonischemic situation, the predominance of the adrenergic response to epinephrine or sympathetic nerve stimulation of the ischemic area is mediated by alpha adrenoceptors. It has been established that the beta adrenergic stimulatory response in the heart is associated with cyclic adenosine monophosphate accumulation which is not involved during alpha stimulation (Wollenberger, 1975). It is tempting to speculate that the physiologic significance of the double mechanism of adrenergic action may be to maintain the responsiveness of the mammalian myocardial muscle under conditions which do not favor a high expenditure of energy.

Our observations that the ischemic myocardium is still able to generate tension and that this preserved contractility can be influenced by inotropic interventions including adrenergic stimuli, are consistent with previous observations by others (Hood et al., 1969; Schelbert et al., 1971; Banka et al., 1975). Collateral coronary blood flow, the average resting level of which has been reported to be as high as 25 to 30% of the normal blood flow in the canine heart was expected to maintain a limited oxygen supply to the ischemic zone throughout the experiments (Schaper, 1971). The level of collateral blood supply is, however, too low to meet even the resting metabolic requirement of the cardiac muscle. Thus, the contractile force generated by the ischemic area must be associated with a considerably reduced myocardial oxydative metabolism.

Recent observations indicated the dependence of cardiac adrenoceptor characteristics on the level of tissue metabolism. The characteristics of these receptors were found to be changed from beta to alpha when decreasing the ambient temperature (Kunos and Szentiványi, 1968.). Similarly, qualitative changes were induced in the coronary (Szentiványi et al., 1970a) and other vascular adrenoceptors (Szentiványi, et al., 1970b) by modifying the metabolic rate of the surrounding tissue, the preponderance of the alpha state being characteristic for the lower, and the preponderance of the beta state for the higher metabolic level. A close functional and morphological association of alpha and beta adrenoceptors has also been established by determining the tissue uptake of their respective antagonists under various experimental circumstances. It was suggested that alpha and beta adrenoceptors represent allosteric conformations of the same structure (Kunos and Nickerson, 1976).

Although the present findings do not prove directly the interconversion of alpha and beta adrenoceptors in the myocardium, their impact is in complete agreement with the above observations. Moreover, the close parallelism between the behavior of myocardial and coronary adrenoceptors provides a further support for this hypothesis. Although the canine coronaries are richly innervated by sympathetic fibers mediating adrenergic alpha vasoconstrictor responses (Juhász-Nagy and Szentiványi, 1971) their normal vasomotor response to adrenergic stimulation is dominated by concomitant changes in myocardial metabolism. Strong stimulation of the stellate ganglion or administration of large doses of catecholamines also increases cardiac oxygen consumption and the alpha constrictor effect is invariably masked by the overriding beta vasodilator response. A great body experiments (for references see Feigl, 1975) demonstrated until now the overwhelming effect of beta vasodilator response in the coronary circulation, as well as the existence of alpha vasoconstriction unmasked by beta receptor blockade. Our present results indicate the possibility of demonstrating a phenomenon opposite to the former one: the unmasking of a certain degree of beta adrenergic vasodilation by alpha adrenoceptor blockade.

After phentolamine administration, a moderate potentiation of the beta vasodilator capacity has been observed even in the normal or non-ischemic coronary bed, indicating a slight, but potentially important restricting influence exerted by the alpha vasoconstrictor mechanism over the beta vasodilator effect. Mohrman and Feigl (1968) have recently demonstrated a similar attenuating influence of alpha-adrenergic vasoconstrictor fibres on coronary vasodilation induced by simultaneous beta-activation. In the presence of alpha-adrenergic blockade they found an augmented flow increase, the potentation amounting to about 30% of the total response. After exposing a selected region of the left ventricle to prolonged acute myocardial ischemia, this potentiation has been found to be significantly exaggerated in our present experiments, the phenomenon being mainly due to an enhanced alpha sensitivity and restricted or lacking beta vasodilator capacity (Figs. 5 and 6). It may be assumed, therefore, that the increased unmasking influence of alpha blockade in association with the decreased beta vasodilator responsiveness of the post-ischemic coronary vessels reflects the diminished metabolic rate induced by prolonged myocardial ischemia. It has been demonstrated that even shorter periods (less than 20 min) of temporary myocardial ischemia induce pronounced damages in regional myocardial metabolism and activity persisting after restoration of the normal blood supply (Weiner et al., 1976). This evidence, completed with the conclusions of the present study, suggests the consideration of the employment of alpha blocking agents in the treatment of some cases of transient cardiac ischemia.

Summary

The effects of acute segmental myocardial ischemia on the characteristics of adrenoceptors mediating inotropic and coronary vascular
responses were studied in open-chest dogs anesthetized with pentobarbital. Epinephrine (0.2 - 0.8 μg/kg i.v.) or supramaximal sympathetic nerve stimulation elicited nearly identical percent increases of
contractile force in both normal and ischemic regions. Phentolamine
(0.5 mg/kg i.v.) significantly reduced adrenergic inotropic responses
in the ischemic area, while those of the normal area were practically
unaffected. In another series of experiments, the adrenergic reactivity
of the coronary blood vessels was studied <u>after</u> release of a prolonged
(1 to 1 - 1/4 hour) period of coronary occlusion. In the post-ischemic
coronary circulation, pharmacologic and nervous adrenergic stimuli induced considerably less vasodilatory reactions than in the control normal bed. Blockade of alpha adrenoceptors by phentolamine significantly
increased the vasodilator capacity of adrenergic stimuli in the post-
ischemic bed, but only slightly increased the adrenergic vasodilator
capacity in the normal coronaries. It was concluded that myocardial
ischemia increases the role played by the myocardial excitatory and
coronary vasoconstrictor alpha adrenoceptors in the heart.

References

Ahlquist, R. P.: A study of the adrenotropic receptors. Am. J. Physiol.
<u>153</u>: 586-599, 1948.

Amsler, G.: Über inverse Adrenalinwirkung. Pfluegers Archiv Gesamte
Physiol. Menschen Tiere <u>185</u>: 86-92, 1920.

Banka, V. S., Bodenheimer, M. H. and Helfant, R. H.: Nitroglycerin
in experimental myocardial infarction. Effect of regional left ventricular length and tension. Am. J. Cardiol. <u>36</u>: 453-458, 1975.

Benfey, B. G.: Characterization of alpha-adrenoceptors in the myocardium. Br. J. Pharmacol. <u>48</u>: 132-138, 1973.

Cotten, M. de V., Moran, N. C. and Stopp, P. E.: A comparison of
the effectiveness of adrenergic blocking drugs in inhibiting the cardiac actions of sympathomimetic amines. J. Pharmacol. Exp. Ther.
<u>121</u>: 183-190, 1957.

Cotten, M. de V. and Walton, R. P.: Dibenamine blockade as a method
of distinguishing between inotropic actions of epinephrine and dig-
italis. Proc. Soc. Exp. Biol. Med. <u>78</u>: 810-815, 1951.

Dale, H. H.: Some physiologic actions of ergot. J. Physiol. (Lond.)
<u>34</u>: 163-206, 1906.

258

Feigl, E. O.: Control of myocardial oxygen tension by sympathetic coronary vasoconstriction in the dog. Circ. Res. 37: 88-95, 1975.

Govier, W. C.: Myocardial alpha receptors and their role in the production of positive inotropic effect by sympathomimetic agents. J. Pharmacol. Exp. Ther. 159: 82-90, 1968.

Govier, W. C., Musal, N. C., Whittington, P. and Broom, A.: Myocardial alpha and beta adrenergic receptors as demonstrated by atrial functional refractory-period changes. J. Pharmacol. Exp. Ther. 154: 255-263, 1966.

Hood, J. R., Covelli, V. H. and Abelman, W. H.: Persistance of contractile behavior in acutely ischemic myocardium. Cardiovasc. Res. 3: 249-260, 1969.

Juhász-Nagy, A. and Kudász, J.: Time-dependent changes of collateral coronary reactivity in the dog. In The Metabolism of Contraction, ed. by P. E. Roy and G. Rona, pp. 483-490, University Park Press, Baltimore, 1975.

Juhász-Nagy, A., Szentiványi, M. and Grosz, G.: Effect of adrenergic activation on collateral coronary blood flow. Jpn. Heart J. 15: 290-299, 1974.

Juhász-Nagy, A. and Szentiványi, M.: Separation of cardioaccelerator and coronary vasomotor fibers in the dog. Am. J. Physiol. 200: 125-129, 1961.

Kunos, G. and Nickerson, M.: Temperature-induced interoconversion of alpha- and beta-adrenoceptors in the frog heart. J. Physiol. (Lond.) 256: 23-40, 1976.

Kunos, G. and Szentiványi, M.: Evidence favoring the existence of a single adrenergic receptor. Nature 217: 1077-1078, 1968.

Mohrman, D. E. and Feigl, E. O.: Competition between sympathetic vasoconstriction and metabolic vasodilation in the canine coronary circulation. Circ. Res. 42: 79-86, 1978.

Moran, N.C. and Perkins, M. E.: An evaluation of adrenergic blockade of the mammalian heart. J. Pharmacol. Exp. Ther. 131: 192-201, 1961.

Newman, W. H.: The influence of drug-induced alterations in the pressor-inotropic state on left ventricular dynamics. Proc. Soc. Exp. Biol. Med. 151: 7-11, 1976.

Nickerson, M. and Chan, G. C. M.: Blockade of responses of isolated
    myocardium to epinephrine. J. Pharmacol. Exp. Ther. _133:_
    186-191, 1961.

Nickerson, M. and Nomaguchi, G. M.: Blockade of epinephrine-induced
    cardioacceleration in the frog. Am. J. Physiol. _163:_ 484-504, 1950.

Schaper, W.: The Collateral Circulation of the Heart, North-Holland,
    Amsterdam, 1971.

Schelbert, J. R., Covell, J. W., Burns, J. W., Maroko, P. R. and
    Ross, J., Jr.: Observations on factors affecting locas forces in
    the left ventricular wall during acute myocardial ischemia. Circ.
    Res. _29:_ 306-316, 1971.

Szentiványi, M., Kunos, G. and Juhász-Nagy, A.: The adrenergic
    reactions of the coronaries in view of a new hypothesis of re-
    ceptors. Acta Physiol. Acad. Sci. Hung. _37:_ 427-428, 1970a.

Szentiványi, M., Kunos, G. and Juhász-Nagy, A.: Modulator theory of
    adrenergic receptor mechanism: vessels of the dog hindlimb. Am.
    J. Physiol. _218:_ 869-875, 1970b.

Wagner, J., Endoh, M. and Reinhardt, D.: Stimulation by phenyl-
    ephrine of adrenergic alpha- and beta-receptors in the isolated
    perfused rabbit heart. Naunyn-Schmiedebergs Arch. Pharmakol.
    _282:_ 307-310, 1974.

Weiner, J. M., Apstein, C. S., Arthur, J. H., Pizarda, F. A. and
    Hood, W. B., Jr.: Persistence of myocardial injury following
    brief periods of coronary occlusion. Cardiovasc. Res. _10:_ 678-686,
    1976.

Wenzel, D. G. and Su, J. L.: Interaction between sympathomimetic
    amines and blocking agents on rat ventricle strip. Arch. Int.
    Pharmacodyn. Ther. _160:_ 379-389, 1966.

Wollenberger, A.: The role fo cyclic AMP in the adrenergic control
    of the heart. _In_ Contraction and Relation in the Myocardium, ed.
    by W. G. Nayler, pp. 113-190, Academic Press, London, 1975.

Discussion

<u>Szentiványi</u>: If your explanation for the shift of alpha/beta balanace after ischemia is correct, one would expect some signs of it to be revealed by more "natural" forms of sympathetic excitation than administration of catecholamines in great doses.

<u>Juhász-Nagy</u>: I would like to comment on this point. After the conclusion of the above collaborative work with Dr. Aviado, we performed other studies in this field.

In accordance with your suggestion, we were able to demonstrate in recent experiments that after subjecting the heart to temporary ischaemia the coronaries are increasingly susceptible to alpha-adrenoceptor regulatory influences. It is know that the decrease of impulse traffic of the carotid sinus baroreceptor afferents causes reflex coronary vasoconstriction and <u>vice versa</u>. Since, under ordinary circumstances this vasoconstriction is accompanied by an increased myocardial stimulation and tachycardia as well, the concomitant beta-adrenoceptor stimulation masks the pure vasomotor control causing the net effect of vasodilation. In the record I show, as an example, between

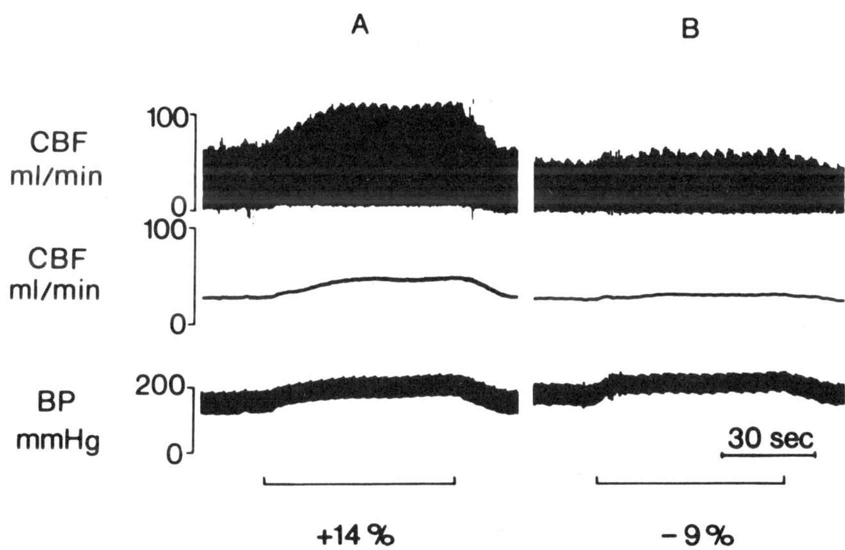

<u>Fig</u>: From above downwards: phasic and mean coronary blood flow, blood pressure. └──┘ Carotid clamping. Percent changes of end-diastolic coronary conductance are also indicated.

A and B a coronary occlusion of 60 min duration was effected.
In A occlusion of both common carotids, a procedure wide-
spreadly used to decrease carotid sinus baroreceptor loading,
induced hypertension, coronary flow increase and a small
augmentation of end-diastolic coronary vascular conductance.
Panel B was taken after release of the LAD artery just
after the coronary flow has been recovered from reactive
hyperemia. Instead of an increase, a decrease of the end-diastolic vascular conductance could be observed on clamping
the carotids, The whole pattern is very similar to that
occuring in beta-adrenergic blockade. In fact, if you like it,
the sensitization of the alpha-adrenergic component of the
reflexarc could be considered a functional beta-blockade
produced by prolonged ischemia.

INDEX

The page numbers refer to the first page of the article in which the index term appears.